Hereditary Malignant Melanoma

Editors

Henry T. Lynch, M.D.
Professor and Chairman
Department of Preventive Medicine and Public Health
Professor of Medicine
Creighton University School of Medicine
Omaha, Nebraska

Ramon M. Fusaro, M.D., Ph.D.
Professor of Dermatology
Department of Medicine
Creighton University School of Medicine
and the University of Nebraska College of Medicine
Professor, Department of Preventive Medicine and Public Health
Creighton University School of Medicine
Omaha, Nebraska

CRC Press, Inc.
Boca Raton Ann Arbor Boston

Library of Congress Cataloging-in-Publication Data

Hereditary malignant melanoma / [editors] Henry T. Lynch, Ramon M. Fusaro.
p. cm.
Includes bibliographical references and index.
ISBN 0-8493-6051-X
1. Melanoma—Genetic aspects. 2. Melanoma—Molecular aspects.
I. Lynch, Henry T. II. Fusaro, Ramon M.
[DNLM: 1. Dysplastic Nevus Syndrome. 2. Melanoma—genetics.
QZ 200 H542]
RC280.M37H47 1991
616.99'477071—dc20
DNLM/DLC
for Library of Congress 90-15143
CIP

Direct all inquiries to CRC Press, Inc., 2000 Corporate Blvd., N.W., Boca Raton, Florida 33431.

International Standard Book Number 0-8493-6051-X

Library of Congress Card Number 90-15143
Printed in the United States

FOREWORD

The incidence of melanoma appears to be rising worldwide. About one-tenth of all melanomas have been estimated to occur in families with hereditary predisposition to this malignancy. Thus, investigations of such families may help to understand the etiology of malignant melanoma and contribute to its early detection. The present volume supplies cogent and timely reviews in this area and will serve as a source of crucial information for those studing these syndromes.

The contents of a book usually speaks for itself. Only rarely does the reader look at or peruse a Foreword, which usually speaks in positive terms of the authors and the volume. This is natural, since authors usually invite a person well acquainted with and favorably predisposed to the area being presented in a book, or a personal friend who has known and shared the apogees and nadirs of their work and studies. I presume that I fall into the latter category.

Over the years, Henry Lynch and Ramon Fusaro have devoted much of their investigative energy in a dogged pursuit of information on the nature of hereditary or familial cancers, and of melanotic lesions in particular. No corner of the U.S. was free of their search for and inquiry into these syndromes; no aspect of these syndromes was too small for their attention and investigation and no stone was left unturned in their persistent examination of the clinical and genetic aspects of these states. We all build on the foundations of others and the work of Lynch and Fusaro is no exception; however, the edifice they have put up is very tall and magnificent. Undoubtedly, the investigation of human malignant melanoma will go on for a long time and in this endeavor the contributions of Lynch and Fusaro on the hereditary aspects of this disease will make this very difficult path much easier.

I wish to congratulate the Editors of this volume not only on their contributions, but also for having selected outstanding experts in this field as contributors to this important book.

I would like to take this opportunity to acknowledge the longstanding friendship I've shared with the authors and the excitement of the many meetings and discussions held and collaborative studies undertaken over these years. I wish them well in this undertaking.

Avery A. Sandberg, M.D., D.Sc.
Scottsdale, Arizona

PREFACE

In the past, the occurrence of cancer in a patient elicited little or no concern about genetic risk implications for the patient's immediate family let alone the kindred. This situation has changed within the last two decades as evidenced by a marked increase in the number and variety of reports of familial cancer aggregations with a new interest in cancer genetics. This interest has become intensified by advances in molecular genetics, by the identification of tumor suppressor genes and their actual cloning (e.g., retinoblastoma gene).

The clearly defined hereditary cancer-prone syndromes now confronting physicians number into the hundreds. We conservatively estimate that at least 5% and possibly as much as 10% of *all* cancers occur in families harboring a major gene for cancer susceptibility. Given these facts, it is paradoxical that a significant hiatus exists between the extant genetic knowledge of cancer and its application to patients and their families in the clinical practice of medicine.

The lack of clinical application of our knowledge of hereditary cancer has many causes. Primary has been the paucity of physicians' knowledge about cancer genetics. Prior to 1970, hereditary cancer problems were only superficially mentioned in the medical literature and were rarely discussed in depth in a medical school curriculum. They could be counted on the fingers of one hand! Undoubtedly, much of the lack of progress in familial cancer care emanates from the fact that a well-executed family cancer history is the most severely neglected portion of the medical evaluation of patients. In addition, patients have invariably little accurate health information of even their immediate family let alone their extended kindred members. The gathering of family cancer information has been further complicated by the medical/legal and ethical issues of confidentiality which inhibits the search for pertinent facts needed to compile an informative status of cancer risks for the kindred. The process is further complicated by the fears and taboos of our personal and cultural concepts of cancer. However, the most serious inhibition is the growing economic penalty of hereditary cancer diagnosis, treatment, and surveillance in high risk kindreds which have been imposed, albeit overtly or occasionally covertly, by institutional health programs and the health insurance industry. Their main goals are promulgated by economic necessity in budgetary limitations and corporate profitability. Hence these actions have developed into a crisis in the care of families with genetic cancer. Within this complicated health care setting, the dedicated physician who institutes cancer genetic studies in a cancer prone family has little incentive for reimbursement for his costs let alone rewards for his efforts; in fact, if he discovers a family with genetic cancer, he has relegated them and their progeny often to the ranks of the uninsurable in the U.S. In other parts of the world under socialized systems of health care, there is little inclination for such pursuits as physicians have to take on extra work loads with minimal or no budgetary incentives or help. Collectively, these negative barriers have imposed a deterrent effect on the development of effective programs for health care of families with hereditary cancer syndromes.

Our book focuses only on hereditary malignant melanoma. The epidemic of cutaneous malignant melanoma which is now occurring in the sun belt areas of the world is due partly to a susceptible subgroup of Caucasians who have immigrated there. We wonder why only a relatively small subset of these Caucasians develop cutaneous malignant melanoma after prolonged exposure to sunlight. Our concepts of the beneficial and detrimental aspects of our environment have changed profoundly in the last 40 years and especially in the last decade. Logically, this led to the study of host factors to explain susceptiblity and resistance to malignant melanoma.

This book is the first treatise dealing with the genetics of malignant melanoma in humans. When we conceived this book, we considered a multidisciplined approach embodying malignant melanoma, beginning at a more primitive infrahuman level (fish, with well-defined melanoma studies) followed by a discussion of the melanoma-associated genetic syndromes, basic immunology, pathology of dysplastic nevi, and a highly detailed description of the genetics of the familial atypical multiple mole melanoma (FAMMM) syndrome. It would appear that the FAMMM or hereditary dysplastic nevus syndrome and its sporadic component may be quantitatively, in the public health sense, the single most important consideration in hereditary malignant melanoma. The FAMMM syndrome for perspective purposes has been described in the context and perspective of other hereditary forms of malignant melanoma. Controversial areas of this cancer associated genodermatosis have been enumerated in order to alert the reader of the unsettled questions of this disorder and the research that is yet to be done in order to significantly improve cancer control in a cost-effective manner.

Investigation into the FAMMM syndrome and its hereditary counterparts has provided many new insights into the genetic etiology of malignant melanoma. It has also promulgated interest into basic carcinogenic and etiological hypotheses for this heterogeneous disease. It is anticipated that research into the FAMMM syndrome may provide insight into the epidemic of malignant melanoma that is now occurring throughout the world particularly in the Caucasian populations residing in the world's "sun belts". It is hoped that the results of this research will lead to public health measures which will be practical and cost effective, thereby curtailing this recent epidemic of malignant melanoma.

THE EDITORS

Henry T. Lynch, M.D., is Professor and Chairman of the Department of Preventive Medicine and Public Health and Professor of Medicine at Creighton University School of Medicine. He is President of Creighton's Hereditary Cancer Institute and Director of the Hereditary Cancer Consultation Center. He is a graduate of the University of Oklahoma (B.S.) and Denver University (M.A. in Clinical Psychology); has done work toward his Ph.D. in genetics, and then entered medical school at the University of Texas Medical Branch, Galveston (M.D. 1960). He completed a residency in Internal Medicine, followed by a two-year fellowship in medical oncology at the University of Nebraska College of Medicine, Omaha. He is a member of Alpha Omega Alpha, Honor Medical Society, a winner of the Billings Silver Medal from the American Medical Association (1966), the Distinguished Service Award from Creighton University (1985), and the Ungerman-Lubin Lecture Prize for Outstanding Cancer Research (1987). Dr. Lynch has published more than 300 scientific papers and 11 books. The majority of these have related to cancer genetics. He was a short-term consultant in oncology to the World Health Organization, and is a consultant to and has been a member of several study groups at the National Cancer Institute. He is currently a consultant to the Food and Drug Administration. His most current book is *Genetic Epidemiology of Cancer,* published by CRC Press in 1989.

Ramon M. Fusaro, M.D., Ph.D., is Chief of the Section of Dermatology, Department of Internal Medicine, and Professor of Preventive Medicine, Creighton University School of Medicine. He is also Professor of Dermatology, Section of Dermatology, Department of Internal Medicine, University of Nebraska Medical Center, Omaha.

Dr. Fusaro graduated from the University of Minnesota, where he received a B.A. (1949), a B.S. (1951), an M.D. (1953), an M.S. (1958), and a Ph.D. (1965). He took his residency training in Dermatology at Minneapolis General Hospital and the University of Minnesota Hospitals (1954—1957) and was a National Cancer Institute trainee (1956—1957). He was board certified by the American Board of Dermatology in July 1959. He was the first full-time faculty member in the Department of Dermatology, University of Minnesota Medical School, as an Associate Professor and Chief of outpatient dermatology clinics. In 1970 he became Chairman of Dermatology at both departments of dermatology at Creighton University Medical School and the University of Nebraska Medical Center.

Dr. Fusaro is a member of the American Academy of Dermatology, Society of Investigative Dematology, American Society for Photobiology, Association of Professors of Dermatology, Dermatology Foundation, International Society of Tropical Dermatology, Hennepin County (Minnesota) Medical Society, and Missouri Valley Dermatological Society.

His present active fields of research include hereditary malignant melanoma, hereditary polymorphic light eruption of American Indians, and sun screens. He has published over 200 scientific publications in 51 national and international scientific journals. He has written chapters or sections in 14 published books and has edited two books. He has received six scientific awards for scientific medical exhibits.

CONTRIBUTORS

Fritz Anders, Ph.D.
Genetics Institute
Justus Liebig University
Giessen, Germany

Dr. Angelika Barnekow
Department of Experimental Tumor Biology
University Muenster
Muenster, Germany

Wilma Bergman, M.D., Ph.D.
Department of Dermatology
University Medical Center
Leiden, The Netherlands

Ian Michael Bird, Ph.D.
Department of Clinical Chemistry
The Royal Infirmary
Edinburgh, United Kingdom

Florence M. Demenais, M.D.
Division of Biostatistics
Howard University Cancer Center
Washington, D.C.

Soldano Ferrone, M.D.
Department of Microbiology and Immunology
New York Medical College
Valhalla, New York

Ramon M. Fusaro, M.D., Ph.D.
Professor of Dermatology
Creighton University School of Medicine
University of Nebraska
Omaha, Nebraska

Lloyd H. Graf, Jr., M.D.
Center for Research in Periodontal Disease and Department of Physiology and Biophysics
University of Illinois
Chicago, Illinois

Dr. Thomas Gronau
Genetics Institute
Justus Liebig University
Giessen, Germany

A. van Haeringen, M.D.
Department of Clinical Genetics
University Medical Center
Leiden, The Netherlands

S. C. Henzen-Logmans, M.D.
Daniel der Koed Cancer Institute
Rotterdam, The Netherlands

Lavonne Johnsen
Research Assistant
Department of Medicine-Dermatology
Creighton University School of Medicine
Omaha, Nebraska

Patricia Ann Lane
Department of Chemical Pathology
University College and Middlesex School of Medicine
London, United Kingdom

Henry T. Lynch, M.D.
Professor and Chairman of Preventive Medicine and Public Health
Creighton University School of Medicine
University of Nebraska
Omaha, Nebraska

Jane F. Lynch, R.N.
Department of Preventive Medicine/Public Health
Creighton University School of Medicine
Omaha, Nebraska

W. J. Mooi, M.D.
Department of Pathology
The Netherlands Cancer Institute
Amsterdam, The Netherlands

Jendo A. Oosterhuis, M.D.
Department of Ophthalmology
University Medical Center
Leiden, The Netherlands

Andre Pröfrock, Dipl. Biol.
Genetics Institute
University of Giessen
Giessen, Germany

Dirk J. Ruiter, M.D.
Department of Pathology
University Hospital
Nijmegen, The Netherlands

E. Scheffer, M.D.
Department of Pathology
University Hospital
Leiden, The Netherlands

A. D. Smith, Ph.D.
Department of Chemical Pathology
University College and Middlesex School of Medicine
London, United Kingdom

P. M. Steylen, M.D.
Department of Dermatology
University Hospital
Nijmengen, The Netherlands

J. Van der Wiel-Miezenbeek, M.D.
Department of Pathology
University Hospital
Nijmengen, The Netherlands

A. Van Haeringen, M.D.
Department of Clinical Genetics
University Medical Center
Leiden, The Netherlands

Loe N. Went, D.Sc.
Department of Human Genetics
University Medical Center
Leiden, The Netherlands

Dr. Christina Zechel
Genetics Institute
Justus Liebig University
Giessen, Germany

ACKNOWLEDGMENTS

This book is dedicated to our wives, Jane and Lavonne, to our Creighton University Medical School, and to our countless patients who participated in this research. Without their help and backing, this book would not have been possible.

TABLE OF CONTENTS

Chapter 1

HEREDITARY MALIGNANT MELANOMA AND THE FAMMM SYNDROME

Henry T. Lynch, Ramon M. Fusaro, Lavonne Johnsen, and Jane F. Lynch

TABLE OF CONTENTS

I. INTRODUCTION

Cutaneous malignant melanoma (CMM) in the U.S. is now increasing in occurrence at a rate second only to lung cancer in women. By the year 2000 A.D., it is estimated that 1 in 100 Caucasians will develop CMM during their lifetime.[1] The cause for this change within the last 3 to 4 decades is multifold: (1) the presence of a genetically susceptible Caucasian population with probable multiple inheritable traits which have been present for eons but are only now being quantitatively activated by geographic, environmental, and social factors; (2) the increasing number of Caucasians who are moving into the sunny climates around the globe (e.g., southern U.S. or Australia); (3) increase in leisure time available for outdoor recreational activity during prime sunlight hours because of affluence and a shorter work week; (4) the wearing of minimal clothing during these activities so that maximum athletic function can be accomplished (little attention is given by manufacturer to protect wearer from exposure to sunlight); (5) exposure to sunlight starting at an *early* age (the first decade) and continuing well into middle adult life; (6) the history of repeated moderate to severe ''sunburns,'' prepubertally; (7) the successful indoctrination of the public by commercial enterprises on the value of prolonged outdoor recreational activities; (8) failure of the medical and paramedical professions to successfully educate the public on the long-term effects of excessive sunlight exposure and need for reduction of outdoor recreational activities during the midday period; and (9) failure of public to use sun screen effectively. These events have led to an increase in sunlight exposure by the general public that is a relatively new, unprecedented experience for Caucasians.

In light of these facts, it is extremely important to realize that *all* individuals who are excessively *exposed* are *not* equal with respect to cancer susceptibility from solar radiation. Some are more susceptible to CMM than others. These differences in susceptibility to CMM result primarily from host factor variation. Those genotypic factors which endow many in our population with fair complexion, blond or red hair, freckles, blue eyes, and poor tanning ability are also extremely important etiologic factors, particularly when they interact with solar radiation. Collectively, these help to explain the enormous upswing in CMM. A less frequent but potentially devastating etiologic factor to specific families is that of Mendelian inheritance of a single deleterious CMM-predisposing gene. Families in which these CMM-prone genes segregate in accord with Mendelian inheritance patterns include the autosomal recessive disorders of albinism and xeroderma pigmentosum. The newly discovered, autosomal dominantly inherited, familial atypical multiple mole melanoma (FAMMM) syndrome (or hereditary dysplastic nevus syndrome [HDNS]) is by far the most common hereditary CMM-predisposing disorder. Collectively, these genetic disorders provide tremendously interesting models for the study of melanoma's carcinogenesis, as well as its control. Multifactorial factors, as in pigmentation and complexion, and Mendelian inherited predisposing genes will provide the major subject matter for this book.

II. HOW DOES SUNLIGHT INTERACT WITH HOST FACTORS IN MELANOMA CARCINOGENESIS?

Surprisingly, there has been limited investigation of the etiologic role of environmental interaction with host factors in CMM, inclusive of the FAMMM. For example, in spite of the prodigious evidence for the significance of solar radiation exposure in the etiology of CMM, we are not aware of *any* definitive clinical evidence showing the effect of sunlight exposure on atypical nevi (AN) or CMM in the FAMMM.

A study of keen interest toward the understanding of the genetic epidemiology of CMM is that of Roser et al.[2] This investigation pertained to the manner in which genetically enhanced susceptibility to ultraviolet (UV) radiation may play a crucial etiologic role in the

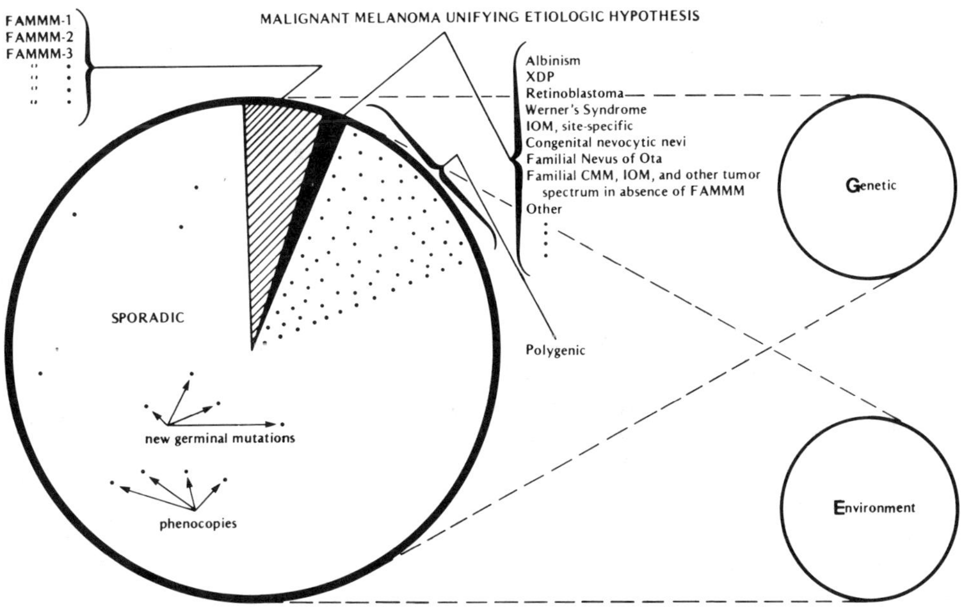

FIGURE 1. The FAMMM syndrome, unifying etiologic hypothesis. FAMMM = familial atypical multiple mole melanoma syndrome (suffixes indicate heterogeneous forms); XDP = xeroderma pigmentosum; IOM = intraocular malignant melanoma, site specific; CMM = cutaneous malignant melanoma. (Reprinted from Lynch, H. T. and Fusaro, R. M., *Cancer Genet. Cytogenet.*, 20, 301, 1986. With permission.)

evolution of CMM at the laboratory level. These researchers studied skin fibroblasts from 26 patients with CMM and controls. They utilized the micronucleus (MN) test and sister chromatid exchange (SCE) following UV radiation. SCE and MN formation were then employed as investigational parameters for the detection of UV-induced genotoxic damage in the individual cell strains. Results disclosed "...that the UV-induced level of MN was significantly increased in CMM patients ($p = 0.0005$), being most pronounced in the familial cases ($p = 0.001$), but there wasn't any difference between familial and nonfamilial cases. The present findings indicate that genetic predisposition contributes to the development of CMM in a subset of CMM patients and may be due to an enhanced susceptibility to UV light." This methodological approach needs to be pursued in well-defined FAMMM kindreds.

III. UNIFYING ETIOLOGY HYPOTHESIS

Lynch and Fusaro[3] proposed a unifying etiologic hypothesis for the etiology of malignant melanoma (see Figure 1). This hypothesis emphasized the occurrence of malignant melanoma as resulting from the interactions of genetics and environment. The hypothesis embraced basic genetic principles of reduced gene penetrance, variable expressivity of the phenotype, and genetic heterogeneity.[4,7] Primary genetic perturbations such as position effects and modifying genes, as well as extragenetic environmental interactions, in concert with such factors as activated oncogenes, may bear directly on melanoma carcinogenesis.[4] Clearly, we are exceedingly low on the learning curve with respect to the identification of the role of primary genetic factors in malignant melanoma. This problem is hampered in a major way by the limited genetic knowledge of many physicians who attend these genetically high risk patients. The problem is seriously confounded: (1) by the fact that the family history is rarely developed in sufficient depth to enable an hereditary cancer syndrome diagnosis; and (2) by variations in clinical expression of phenotype, which may be extant and thereby require detailed clinical and genetic analysis of the patients and their family members.

The following CMM-predisposing disorders, while rare, are nevertheless pertinent to the understanding of the genetics of malignant melanoma, in the context of this hypothesis.

A. ALBINISM

Albinism is a genetic spectrum of disease involving different aspects of the metabolism and distribution of melanin in the skin, hair, and eyes. The term albinism is limited to those congenital universal hypomelanoses that involve the skin and eye (oculocutaneous albinism [OCA]) and the eye alone (ocular albinism [OA]). There are ten types of OCA: (1) tyrosinase-negative (ty-neg) OCA, (2) tyrosinase-positive (ty-pos) OCA, (3) yellow mutant OCA (YMA) (4) plastinum OCA (pt-OCA), (5) Hermansky-Pudlak syndrome (HPS), (6) brown OCA (BA), (7) rufous OCA (RA), (8) Cross-McKusick-Breen syndrome (CMBS), (9) black locks-albinism-deafness syndrome (BADS), and (10) Chediak-Higashi syndrome. The cutaneous findings are an absence or decrease in melanin pigmentation of the skin and hair. The eyes show the same pigmentation changes, but in addition, there is nystagmus, photophobia, and decreased visual acuity. All of these are inherited in an autosomal recessive pattern. At the other end of the genetic spectrum of OCA are the dominant forms with cutaneous hypomelanoses: (1) autosomal dominant OCA and (2) oculocutaneous albinoidism. In addition, there is albinism limited to the eye — ocular albinism. The skin is usually normal in color. There are five types of ocular albinism with only ocular pigmentation abnormalities: (1) X-linked type (Nettleship or Vogt), (2) X-linked type (Forsius-Eriksson or Aland eye disease), (3) Winship type, (4) autosomal recessive ocular albinism, and (5) autosomal dominant ocular albinism.[5]

The cutaneous complications of the OCA are seen in the development of early onset premalignant keratoses and virulent squamous cell carcinoma of the skin which appear to increase in incidence as these patients with OCA live closer to the equator. The development of malignant melanoma (80% are amelanotic melanoma) is an extremely rare complication within this heterogeneous group of disorders. There are only 20 such cases reported. This low number may be due to lack of interest in reporting CMM in the face of the excessive burden of squamous cell carcinoma seen in these patients.[6]

B. XERODERMA PIGMENTOSUM

Xeroderma pigmentosum (XDP) is an exceedingly rare, autosomal recessive, multisystem disorder. The principal target organ is the skin where the manifestations are dependent on age and environment, particularly solar radiation. Pathologic changes in the skin are variable, but include disturbances of pigmentation and maturation of epidermal cells, leading eventually to the formation of malignant skin tumors, usually basal and squamous cell carcinomas. Malignant melanoma appears to have at least a 10% association with this disease, but its incidence will undoubtedly increase as these patients survive for longer periods of time into adulthood.[7]

The pioneering efforts of Cleaver,[8] studying DNA repair defects induced by UV radiation (UVR), stimulated interest in XDP at the molecular level. XDP is more heterogeneous than originally perceived, as evidenced by the presence of at least eight subgroups that are based on the ability to repair DNA after UV irradiation of cultured skin fibroblasts. Cells deficient in excision repair (classic XDP) have been classified as complementation groups A through G; at least one other group, the XDP variant, exhibits defective postreplication repair. Two additional complementation groups, H and I, are questionable; the former was reported as identical with group D[9] and the latter with group C.[10] The XDP cell types seem to be controlled by a separate allele since multiple patients affected within a given kindred show the same complementation group.[11]

We have studied a family with XDP for more than two decades (see Figure 2). Interestingly, five of nine siblings manifested clinically and pathologically verified XDP. During

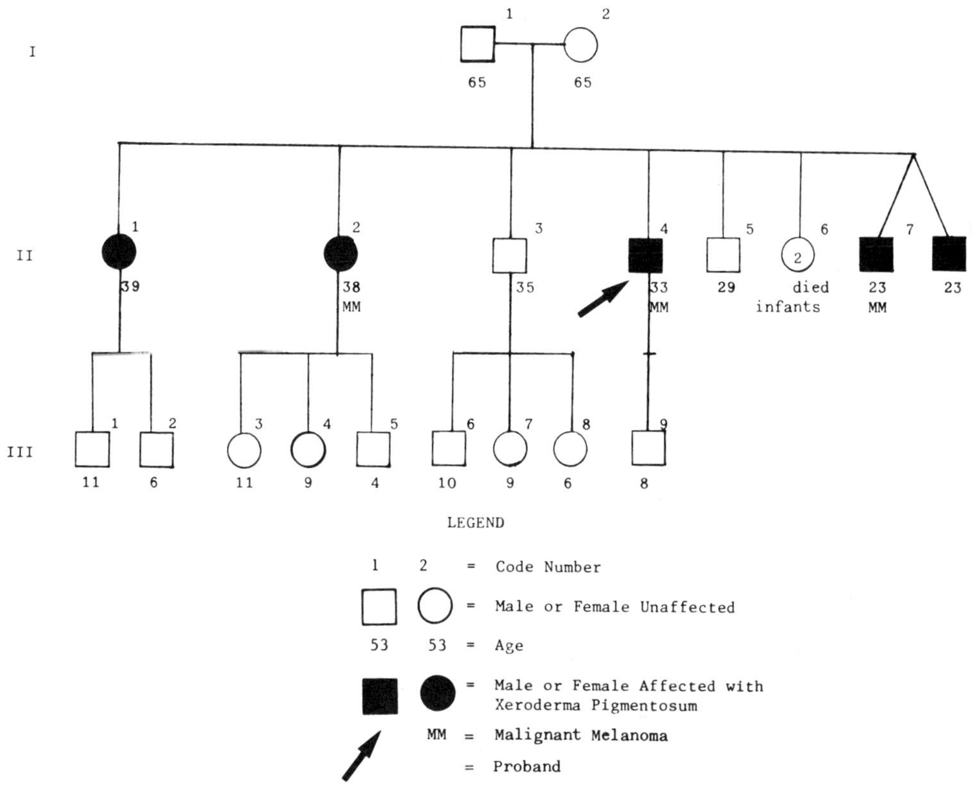

FIGURE 2. XDP pedigree.

the course of this study, two of these patients (see Figure 2, II-2, II-4) developed metastatic malignant melanoma which underwent spontaneous regression.[12] The pathology report of one of these patients showed features of possible spontaneous regression; namely, foamy histiocytes, capillary proliferation, and a chronic inflammatory infiltrate which was devoid of malignant cells, suggesting the possibility that an immunological mechanism was at work.

It was of interest that a review of 27 cases of spontaneous regression of metastatic malignant melanoma since 1900 contained a patient with XDP.[13] Adding our two cases, at least 10% of the spontaneous regressions of metastatic melanoma occurred in patients with XDP. This unusual association raised the question that the genotype for XDP may possibly foster control of metastatic malignant melanoma in some, as yet unknown, way.

We had provided skin samples from this family for fibroblast studies in Cleaver's early investigations on DNA repair. This study disclosed complementation group C to be present in all five XDP-affected members of this kindred. A CMM developed in one of the XDP identical twins (see Figure 2, II-7) since our mentioned study on complementation group C and CMM in XDP. Our literature review[14] showed complementation group C to have occurred in excess association with malignant melanoma in XDP patients.[15] Because of the high frequency of CMM associated with complementation group C, we suggested several possible hypotheses:

1. The association between CMM and XDP is a firm one based on the natural history of XDP, but its putative increased association with complementation group C may be fortuitous.
2. The CMM association with complementation group C may be causative and thereby

indicative of an as yet unknown underlying mechanism that predisposes patients with this XDP complementation group to CMM.

3. Other exogenous or endogenous factors may interact with the XDP gene, leading to CMM susceptibility, in group C patients. This postulate will require more intensive investigation of patients with XDP and complementation group C.
4. Patients with XDP, complementation group C, may have a better chance of survival than patients belonging to the other subgroups, and as a result, live long enough to sustain sufficient carcinogenic exposures (especially to UVR) to increase the probability of having CMM.

C. GIANT PIGMENTED NEVUS

Giant pigmented nevi are present at birth. These nevi are usually greater than 930 cm^2 (or >20 cm in diameter) but individuals can have multiple nevi of small size, usually exceeding 1.5 cm in diameter. The giant lesion can be unilateral, but is usually bilateral and symmetrical. There is a tendency toward dermatome distribution. The pigment is highly variable, but is usually dark brown to black. The lesions can be extremely verrucous and hairy. Growth of the nevi parallels that of the child. The CMM is an important sequelae of this congenital nevus.

These giant nevi may be associated with other external manifestations such as many smaller pigmented nevi, fibromas, lipomas, and cafe-au-lait spots. There is a relationship of importance between large congenital nevi and leptomeningeal melanocytosis with certain neurologic complications (seizures, mental retardation, hydrocephalus), especially if the giant pigmented nevi are present on head or neck.[16-22]

In the vast majority of cases, the giant pigmented nevi occur as an isolated congenital process.[7] We are aware of two reports which mention autosomal dominant inheritance of this lesion.[23,24]

D. RETINOBLASTOMA

Traboulsi et al.[25] described six survivors of bilateral (hereditary) retinoblastoma who developed CMM 20 to 51 years (average 31 years) after they received initial therapy for the ocular tumor. Five of these patients received radiation therapy to the orbital area and, in two of them, CMM occurred in the field of irradiation. Of interest was the fact that two of the patients developed multiple CMMs, and they were thought to manifest the FAMMM. The review of the literature by these authors indicated that CMM accounted for about 7% of second primary cancers in survivors of hereditary retinoblastoma. CMM has been observed to occur in excess among relatives of patients with hereditary retinoblastoma.[26]

IV. HEREDITARY INTRAOCULAR MALIGNANT MELANOMA

Intraocular malignant melanoma (IOM) comprises a relatively small proportion of all varieties of malignant melanoma. However, it is the most common malignant neoplasm of the eye. This lesion occurs most frequently after the 5th and 6th decades of life and is extremely rare in children. It seems to have a definite racial predilection, being most frequently found in Caucasians and rarely in Negroes. This racial difference is reflected by the Registry of Ophthalmic Pathology of the Armed Forces Institute of Pathology, where the ratio of ocular melanoma in Caucasians to non-Caucasians is 250:1.[27] There is no significant difference in frequency in men and women.

The clinical behavior of metastases of this lesion is highly unpredictable. In some patients, the disease may have a fulminant course; in others, as many as 20 or more years may elapse after enucleation of the affected eye before widespread dissemination occurs.[28] The principal site of metastasis is the liver. In some cases, the liver may be the only site of metastasis and, indeed, may seemingly represent a new primary tumor; however, in other patients, virtually every organ and tissue of the body, just as in metastases from cutaneous malignant melanoma, may ultimately be involved with metastatic disease.

The etiology of IOM remains elusive. Several studies[29-35] have suggested an hereditary basis for this lesion in particular families. Lynch et al.[36] and Oosterhuis et al.[37] have described IOM in the FAMMM syndrome, where it is believed to be an integral lesion.[7]

Lynch et al.[38] reviewed the medial records of 45 patients with histologically confirmed IOM and observed only one example of the lesion occurring in a relative. Clearly, the hereditary variant of IOM is rare. In a separately ascertained IOM kindred, Lynch et al.[38] described IOM occurring in the direct line of descent through three generations. IOM in the hereditary setting appears to have an earlier age of onset, a phenomenon which is in common with practically all examples of hereditary cancer.

In summary, our hypothesis mandates environmental interaction with the basic human genetic pool. These environmental effects are influenced by the macromilieu of chemical, physical (particularly sunlight), and nutritional factors, and the micromilieu of biological agents, such as oncogenes and viruses of putative etiologic importance, which act in concert to modify the basic genetic expression of the human disease.[7] Clues to the understanding of this complex hypothesis may be unraveled at the subhuman level (see Chapter 8).

Much work is yet to be accomplished before we can have an adequate comprehension of melanoma genetics, inclusive of the FAMMM. Although we have stressed the importance of monogenic melanoma predisposing diseases, one must also consider the likelihood of polygenic or multifactorial etiology for a substantial proportion of the melanoma burden (see Figure 1). Failure to intensify our efforts in an eclectic manner in the search for knowledge about melanoma genetics will merely perpetuate a narrow concept of hereditary CMM.[39]

V. PROBLEM AREAS IN CANCER GENETICS

Problems which obscure our comprehension of the genetics and natural history of all forms of hereditary cancer in general, including the FAMMM, include: (1) man's long generation intervals; (2) inability to control matings; (3) limited number of progeny; (4) early deaths from unrelated causes of at risk individuals; and (5) difficulty in obtaining definitive clinical and pathologic documentation of specific cancer(s) occurrences. Key relatives may not comply with the investigation, thereby limiting disclosure of vital medical/genetic information. Thus, sorting out some of these rather perplexing medical/genetic/epidemiologic clues, as in the case of FAMMM's diagnosis, requires patient compliance, timeliness of examination, meticulous documentation of genealogical, medical, and pathologic information, and an enormous amount of patience and diligence. In spite of these limitations, there is an unparalleled power for elucidation of etiology and natural history embodied in the retrospective/prospective investigation of the type we have described previously.[7]

VI. HISTORICAL ASPECTS OF HEREDITARY CMM

Norris[40] is credited with what may possibly be the *first* description of a family with the hereditary form of CMM. The description of the cutaneous phenotype in this family may be consistent with the FAMMM syndrome. Melanoma appeared in a 59-year-old male. Thirty years prior to his death, his father died of a similar disease. Reportedly, a surgeon who had attended this patient's father observed that he had many moles on various parts of his body and that his children, including the index patient, also had multiple moles. The surgeon suggested that the disease was hereditary.

There were no further reports of familial malignant melanoma until the contemporary study by Cawley et al.[41] who described CMMs in a father and two of his three children. Subsequently, Lynch et al.[42] and Clark et al.[43] described the FAMMM or HDNS simultaneously in 1978. As mentioned, this disorder has also been termed the hereditary dysplastic nevus syndrome (HDNS), and these terms will be used interchangeably in this chapter. This syndrome is characterized by an autosomal dominantly inherited predisposition to multiple atypical nevi (AN), total body mole counts greater than usual, and cutaneous malignant melanomas. However, as in virtually *all* hereditary disorders, particularly those showing an autosomal dominant inheritance pattern, there is variable expressivity of the phenotype and reduced penetrance of the gene. There are also problems in the interpretation of phenocopies and genocopies. Therefore, any classical, clinical genetic definition, as we have provided, must be tempered by these potentially limiting obfuscations.

VII. TERMINOLOGY

In the paper by Clark et al.,[43] the disorder was initially referred to as the B-K mole syndrome. A litany of names for this disorder(s) has appeared in the literature; e.g., DNS[44] and the large atypical nevus syndrome (LANS),[45] to name just two of these terms. However, Lynch and Fusaro[3] have considered "FAMMM" to be appropriately descriptive of the hereditary syndrome and have steadfastly adhered to this terminology. Interestingly, investigators have now come almost full circle in the matter of nomenclature, as evidenced by the latest suggested terminology; namely, "atypical mole syndrome" (both hereditary and sporadic), as designated by Kopf et al.[46] This latter designation (Atypical Mole Syndrome) does not clearly separate the hereditary from sporadic concepts and places the diagnosis on the pivotal criterion of the histologic confirmation of the clinical presence of the cutaneous AN phenotype. This reliance on only the AN phenotype along with its histologic confirmation for the diagnosis of the FAMMM syndrome may lead to over-diagnosis of the disorder. As will be discussed subsequently, the AN may occur in normal individuals, thereby posing an often vexing diagnostic problem for the *exclusion* of the FAMMM.

VIII. PROTOTYPE CLINICAL/GENETIC MODEL OF THE FAMMM

Our original FAMMM kindred (see Figure 3) has been followed by us for almost a quarter century.[12,36,47-50] This single kindred has provided us with the unique opportunity to extensively study the genetics, pathology, and natural history of the FAMMM (see Table 1). Clearly, the cutaneous phenotype in the proband (see Plate 1*) and its evolution of AN in his daughter (see Plate 2*) depicts these phenotypic findings in high relief. However, during the past decade, we have learned that *variation* in all facets of the phenotypes must be meticulously scrutinized so that the best posits of the clinical and pathologic study can be used for securing confidence in diagnosis.

The proband (see Figure 3, IV-4) is now a 50-year-old white male (he was age 26 when first studied by us) who has a past history of 13 separate primary CMMs. He and his melanoma-prone relatives were initially investigated by Lynch and Krush.[47] Table 1 shows the anatomic sites and ages at onset of CMM in addition to the associated cutaneous phenotype in the proband and his relatives.

Physical examination of the proband showed him to be a well-nourished, well-developed athlete (collegiate swimmer). He did not begin any form of protection of his skin from sunlight until about age 20 (after his *first* CMM diagnosis), and this only included minimal

* Plates 1 and 2 appear following page 30.

TABLE 1
Registry of Melanoma and Cutaneous Phenotypes

Ped. no.	Age of onset	Anatomic site	Atypical moles[b]	Excessive moles (200 or more)	Comments
III-2	47	Abdomen	Yes	Yes	
	56	Back			
III-3	45	Back	Yes	Yes	Died of CMM
IV-4	20	Left arm	Yes	Yes	
	21	Right costal marg.			
	22	Left lateral malleolus			
	24	Right arm			
	25	Midback			dx by HTL
	26	[a]			40 bx in 10 years w/2 CMM
	36	[a]			Total 13 CMM
IV-5	31	Right wrist	Yes	Yes	4 CMM
	32	Right elbow			
	33	Leg			
	34	Back			
IV-6	—		Yes	Yes	No CMM
IV-7	—		Yes	Yes	No CMM
V-1			Yes	Yes	CMM @ 19 Years
V-2			No	No	

[a] CMM — site unknown.
[b] Histologic verification.

protection with a sunscreen. He had red hair, blue eyes, and his light skin was characterized by multiple freckles and moles over all surface areas, with greatest prominence on the skin of the trunk (see Plate 1). The freckling pattern was extensive in sun-exposed areas. The patient had several hundred moles of variable size and many atypical moles of varying color (brown, pink, and red) with irregular borders and pigment leakage.

His sister (IV-5) developed four primary malignant melanomas (histologically verified) of the skin at ages 31 and 32, and two separate CMMs at age 34. Examination of her skin showed freckling and multiple moles (several hundred), some of which were atypical. Her cutaneous phenotype was strikingly similar to her brother, the proband. During our initial physical examination of this patient, we observed a very atypical, reddish-brown mole measuring 0.4 cm. The lesion was excised by her physician and histologically was a superficial spreading malignant melanoma, her fourth separate primary malignant melanoma.

The proband's mother (III-2) had CMM (histologically verified) at ages 47 and 56. She recently died from pancreatic cancer at age 73. Our examination of her skin had revealed multiple moles (>50), with more than 10 AN. She had had many moles removed, with histological confirmation of severe histologic dysplasia. Her sister (III-3) developed CMM at age 45 (histologically verified) and died at age 55. We had not examined her. She had many moles removed prior to 1975. A review of some of these tissue slides revealed histologic architectural dysplasia with cellular atypia, dermal fibrosis, and a chronic lymphocytic infiltrate. A second sister (IV-6) of the proband had several hundred moles with at least 50 AN (greater than 4 mm) (histologic confirmation of several). She developed her first CMM at age 29. A brother (IV-7) had more than 100 moles, with greater than 30 AN which were confirmed histologically to be dysplastic nevi (DN).

The proband's maternal grandfather (II-2) had pancreatic cancer, as did his sister, the proband's maternal great-aunt (II-1). This great-aunt had a daughter (III-1) with CMM. This patient did not have atypical moles, and had less than 30 total normal-appearing nevi.

The proband's daughter (V-1) was first evaluated by us in 1976 when she was age 5

LEGEND FOR FIGURES 3 TO 6

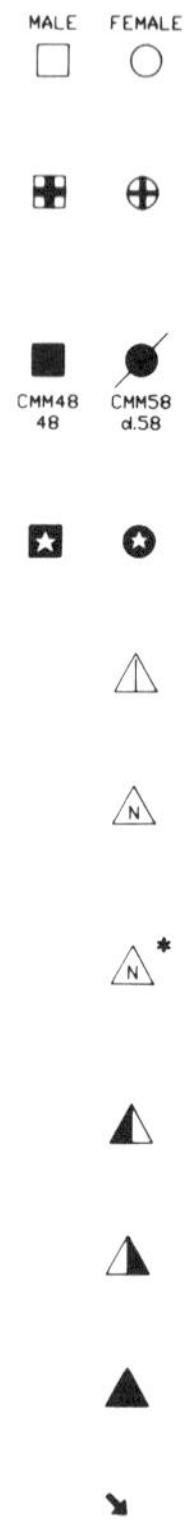

- Unaffected
- Cancer by Death Certificate or Medical Records
- Cancer verified by pathology
- Cancer site and age at diagnosis
- Current age and age at death
- Multiple primary verified by pathology
- History of moles, not previously examined
- Normal/no moles
- Family members nevi examined in 1975; prior to recognition of FAMMM phenotype
- Clinically FAMMM moles
- Histologically FAMMM, not seen clinically
- Clinically and histologically FAMMM
- Proband

Cancer Site

AST	Astrocytoma
BR	Breast
CO	Colon
CMM	Cutaneous malignant melanoma
CSU	Cancer site unknown
CX	Cervix
EN	Endometrium
HO	Hodgkins
IOM	Intraocular melanoma
LU	Lung
LYM	Lymphoma
LYX	Larynx
OV	Ovarian
PAN	Pancreas
PRO	Prostate
ST	Stomach
TON	Tonsil

years. Results of the physical examination of the then 5-year-old child showed an area on her back (see Plate 2A) where there were several small (less than 5 mm) nevi that were uniformly light tan to brown but too small to clearly evaluate clinically. Three years later, her nevi had increased in size and number greater than her proportional growth with respect to height and size. These nevi changed in coloration; some developed pink and brown hues, while others became very dark tan or brown. Some were no longer uniform in coloration and others became papular. One of these lesions in the midback was excised (see Plate 2B*) and found to have histopathologic characteristics consonant with DN with cellular atypia. In addition, a very small macular nevus was noted on the scalp. Her mother had noted the first appearance of these nevi when the child was age 2 years. This observation was of keen interest to us in that the proband's mother also stated that her three FAMMM-affected progeny showed onset of moles at age 2 years.

On her physical examination at age 17 years (see Plate 2C), there was a continued increase in size and number of her nevi. She had greater than 65 total moles, of which 15 were clinically atypical. They now varied markedly in size from a few millimeters up to 15 mm, with irregular borders and leakage of pigmentation. The pigment itself varied from dark brown to light brown to red, and was not distributed uniformly in each nevus. There were some with slightly raised portions and a mottled type of appearance that tended to be darker in color. On the back and rest of the body there were a number of small pigmented lesions that seemed more consistent with normal-appearing moles in that their borders were well defined and pigmentation was uniform. She had on reddish-brown pigmented lesion that measured 1 cm in diameter on the right parietal scalp. This lesion was excised and found to have mild architectural dysplastic changes suggestive of AN.

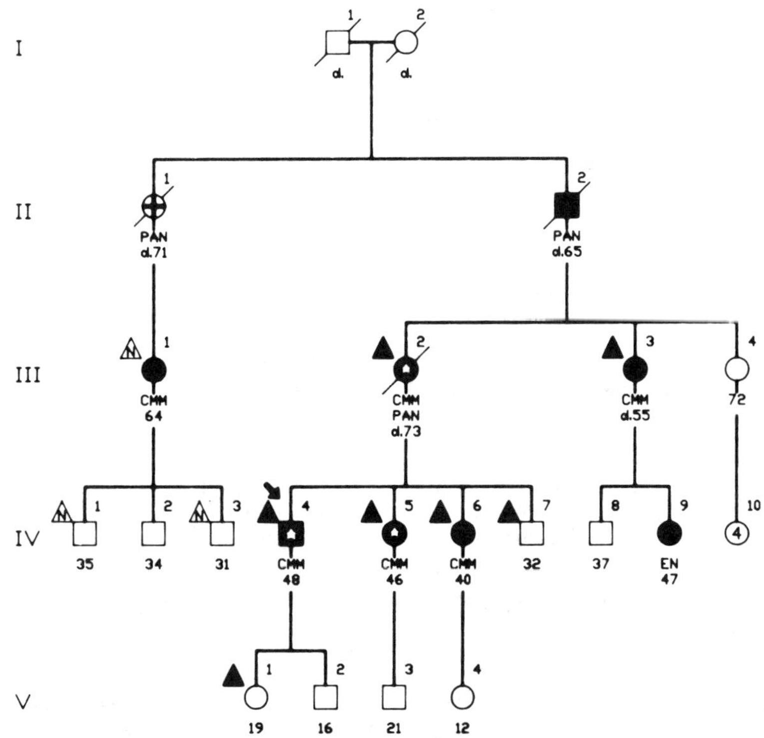

FIGURE 3. This pedigree shows the proband with multiple primary CMMs (13 in over a 25-year period) and occurrence of pancreatic carcinoma in putative obligate gene carriers.

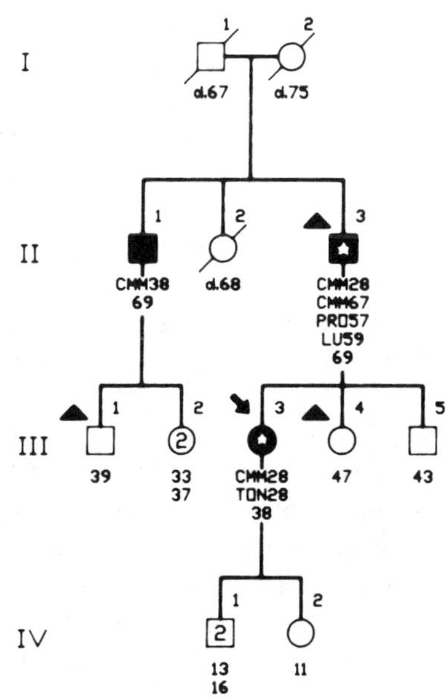

FIGURE 4. Pedigree showing an unusual systemic cancer, tonsillar carcinoma in a young female. (Reprinted from Lynch, H. T. et al., *J. Med. Genet.*, 20, 25, 1983. With permission.)

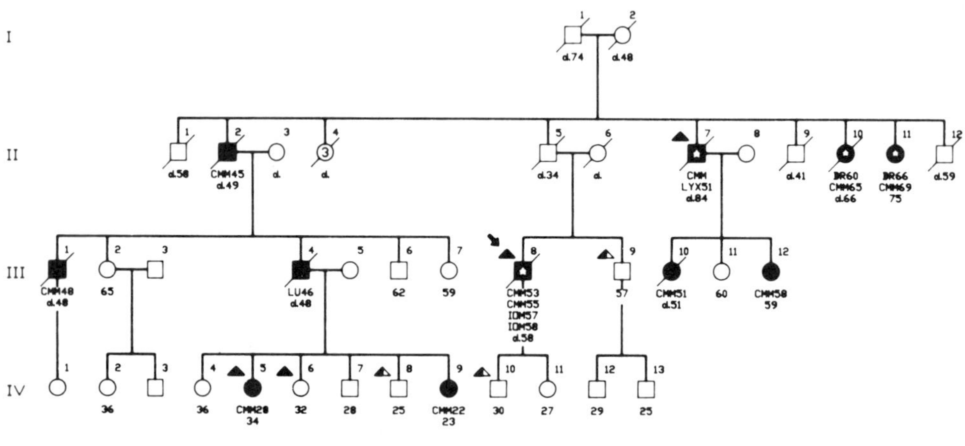

FIGURE 5. Pedigree showing an unusual bilateral intraocular melanoma (IOM) in a member who had multiple cutaneous malignant melanomas (CMMs) and other tumors in obligate gene carrier. (Reprinted from Lynch, H. T. et al., *Br. J. Cancer*, 44, 553, 1981. With permission.)

IX. FAMMM KINDREDS AND SEGREGATION ANALYSIS

In 1983, we studied four of our FAMMM kindreds which showed clinical and pathologic verification of the FAMMM phenotype in multiple family members who had been under our investigation, at that time, for as long as 16 years.[7,36,48,51-53] There were 80 affected or at risk members in these families. Ascertainment of these FAMMM kindreds was made through physician referral or diagnosis of the cutaneous phenotype in probands or both by one of the authors.

A genetic analysis was done to determine the frequency of the FAMMM syndrome among offspring at risk. Using a conservative approach for our analysis, we eliminated all of the probands and their affected parents in the direct line of "ascent". Thus, eight persons were excluded, leaving 72 informative family members who could be included in the genetic analysis. A person was considered affected if he/she had CMM or pathologically verified atypical moles, or both.[7,48] Overall, 34 out of 72 (47%) of the scorable family members conformed to these criteria (see Table 2). No sex differences relative to risk, age of onset, or severity of phenotype were observed. Furthermore, no heterogeneity between families with regard to these same parameters was observed, although the sample is as yet too limited to preclude the possibility of heterogeneity. Consequently, all analyses were done assuming a homogeneous age of onset distribution among all four families. Male-to-male transmission observed in these pedigrees excluded X linkage.

Expressivity of the FAMMM gene with respect to various phenotypic effects among identified and obligate gene carriers was evaluated (see Table 3). For the determination of the phenotypic associations, the total sample of 42 affected family members was used. Those eight family members who were discarded in the previous analysis were therefore included. CMM occurred in 50% and atypical moles in 54% of the gene carriers. Because CMM or pathologically verified atypical moles or both were used as the definition of an affected family member, these estimates are severely biased and represent maximal frequencies. These results do, however, show the variation in the phenotype and underscore the unreliability of complete dependence on the presence of both of these physical findings in a single patient when attempting to establish the diagnosis of the FAMMM syndrome. Three subjects (7.1%) were identified who did not show any manifestation of this disorder, but who were obligate gene carriers on the basis of pedigree analysis (that is, they had affected parents and children). The 7.1% rate of nonpenetrance (92.9% penetrance frequency) must

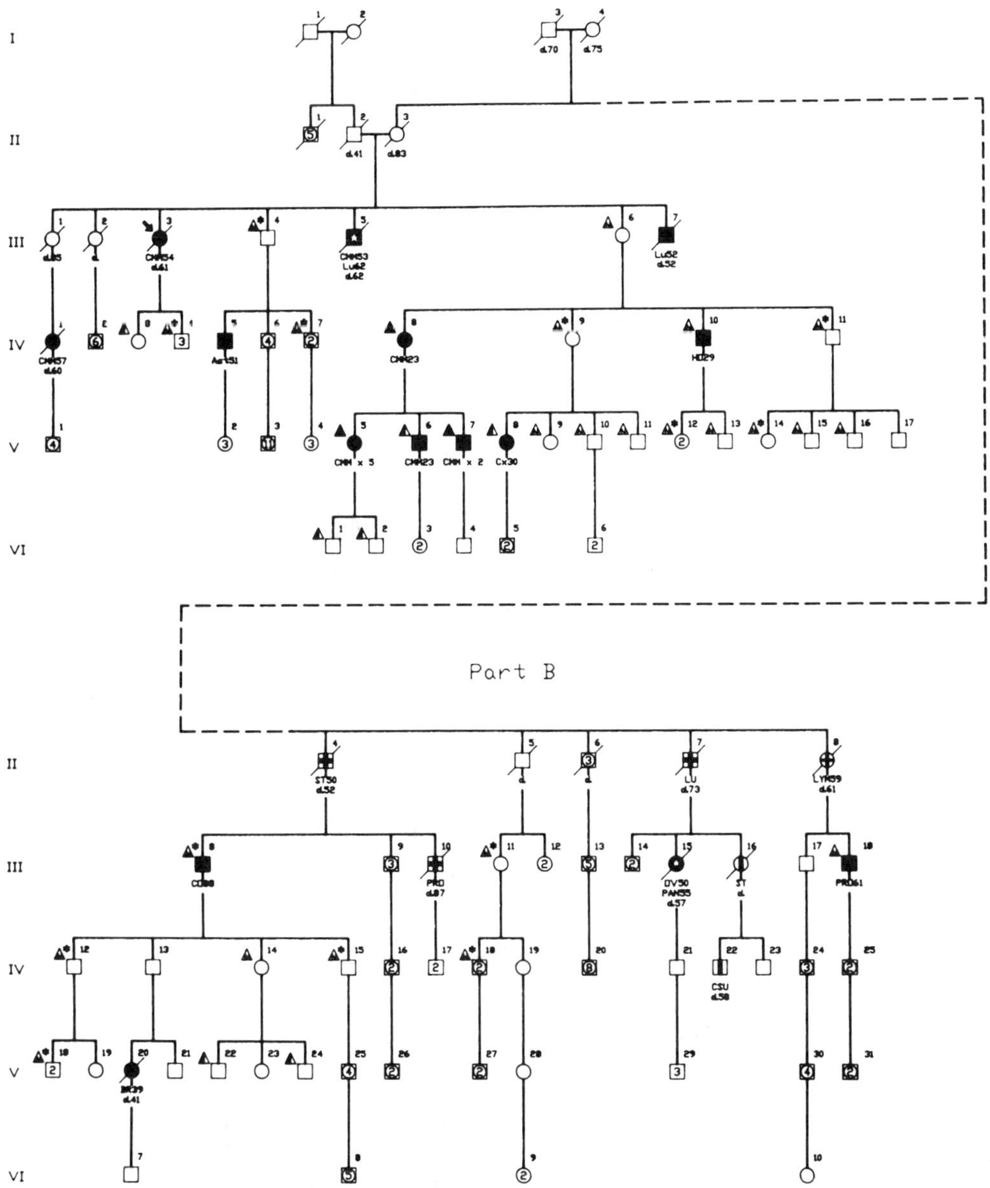

FIGURE 6. Pedigree showing a female member (III-6) with no systemic or cutaneous phenotype and cancer-free at age 70 but by virtue of her position in the pedigree is a putative obligate gene carrier. Since this pedigree was published, individuals V-2 and V-3 have developed CMM. (Reprinted from Lynch, H. T. et al., *Br. J. Cancer*, 44, 58, 1980. With permission.)

be considered minimal inasmuch as it would have been impossible to have detected any unaffected gene carrier who had no affected children. The data were insufficient to calculate an age-specific penetrance rate, and the penetrance rate given here was calculated from the total sample and included family members under the age of 20 years. We would expect that, as more data become available, the penetrance rate would be found to be positively correlated with age.

There appeared to be a strong association of gene carrier status with other neoplasms. This is illustrated in Table 3. Gene carriers show a statistically significant increase in the

TABLE 2
Frequency of Affected by Age Group

Age	Affected	Normal	Total
0—20 years	2	6	8
21—50 years	21	23	44
51 years	11	9	20
Total	34[a]	38	72

Note: Segregation ratio = 34/72 = 0.47.

[a] X^2-test with one degree of freedom was used and the result was not significantly different from 1/2.

TABLE 3
Cancer Table (n = 42 Gene Carriers)

	No. of patients	Observed (%)	Expected[a] (%) (age adjusted)
CMM	21[b]	50.0	—
Atypical nevi	23	54.8	—
No CMM or nevi	3	7.1	—
Lung	3	7.1	0.8 (p <0.02)[c]
Pancreas	2[d]	4.8	0.2 (p <0.02)[c]
Breast	2	4.8	0.6 (p <0.04)[c]
Prostate	1	2.4	—
Tonsil	1	2.4	—
Larynx	1	2.4	—
All non-CMM cancer (all sites)	9[e]	21.4	4.1 (p <0.004)[c]

[a] Cutler, S. J. and Young, J. L., *Natl. Cancer Inst. Monog.*, 411, 1975.
[b] Number of CMM is now 22.
[c] Exact probability of x or more affected calculated using binomial expansion.
[d] One patient had both lung and prostate cancer.
[e] Number of pancreatic adenocarcinomas is now three (see Figure 3, III-2).

incidence of non-CMM cancers. Thus, 9 out of 42 (21% gene carriers have been affected with a cancer other than malignant melanoma. In addition, there is a less striking but still significant increase in the number of patients with cancers of the lung, pancreas, and breast. The mean age of the sample of affected family members is 38 years. Expected values were calculated from data presented in the Third National Cancer Survey[54] and were, of course, age-adjusted.

These data lend statistical support to our hypothesis that the FAMMM syndrome is inherited as an autosomal dominant trait[36,48] and displays variable expressivity and reduced penetrance. While half of our sample of gene carriers developed CMM, the lifetime risk for CMM could be greater and needs to be calculated from a larger sample. There is (Table 3) an increased statistical risk for cancers at *other* anatomic sites. This finding was not unexpected. Specifically, we have found an increased cancer spectrum in the majority of simple, inherited cancer and precancer disorders; for example, ataxia telangiectasia where, in addition to lymphoma and leukemia, sarcomas, squamous cell carcinoma, and epithelial malignancies are observed.[7] If corroborated by additional family data, the management of patients affected with the FAMMM syndrome should be expanded to include surveillance for the presence of these other cancers.

TABLE 4
Tumor Registry of Alabama Kindred

Patient	Sex	Age @ Ca onset	Cancer Dx	Ca site	Verif.	Clin. DN	Histol. DN
II-1	M	38	CMM	Sk	PR	−	−
II-3	M	28	CMM	Sk	PR	+	+
		55	Adeno	Pro	PR		
		59	Sq cell	Lu	PR		
		67	CMM	Sk	PR		
III-1	M					+	+
III-3	F	28	CMM	Sk	PR	−	−
		28	Sq cell	Tons	PR		
III-4	F					+	+

Note: Adeno = adenocarcinoma; Ca = cancer; CMM = cutaneous malignant melanoma; DN = dysplastic nevi; Lu = lung; PR = pathology report; Pro = prostate; Sk = skin; Sq Cell = squamous cell; + = examined, FAMMM nevi; − = examined, normal nevi.

We had previously reported a suspected increased tumor spectrum in the FAMMM based on a single informative kindred.[36] It was therefore of interest that in these four mentioned pedigrees, cancer of *all* anatomic sites combined, excluding CMM and IOM (see Table 3), showed a fivefold increase in risk to gene carriers when age corrected and compared to population expectations. Furthermore, it should be emphasized that cancer, other than CMM, was not a criterion for the diagnosis of gene carrier status. There were other family members who did develop cancer, but who were not counted as gene carriers because they lacked the cutaneous physical findings necessary by our preliminary definition for such a designation.

An increase in risk for non-CMM cancers at "all sites" appears to be supported by these data, but the significance of the apparent increased risk of cancer of the lung, breast, and pancreas is not as secure, as the low numbers of patients relative to the numbers of site-specific cancers makes one wary of a random sampling effect. Consequently, the results relative to specific sites are tentative; however, the occurrences of certain cancers are worthy of note. The occurrence of squamous cell carcinoma of the tonsil in a young (29-year-old) female lacking environmental risk factors (nonalcoholic and essentially nonsmoking) was of unusual interest (see Figure 4, see Table 4 — Alabama).[53] In addition, she had a previous history of CMM without having any atypical moles. Her father had FAMMM moles and developed CMM at the age of 29. Later, he developed two separate primary cancers (lung and prostate) when aged 53 and 56 years, and recently has developed an additional CMM at age 67.

One of the FAMMM kindreds which we studied in Holland (see Figure 5, see Table 5)[36] had a member of the family who had multiple CMMs and later developed (a year apart) two separate primary IOMs. The incidence of CMM and IOM in general population studies has been found to be about 4 in 100,000 and 1 in 100,000, respectively.[54] Hence, the chance of simultaneous but coincidental occurrences of these lesions in the same patient would be practically nil. A review of published reports showed only two FAMMM patients who showed both IOM and CMM[36,37,55] and only 22 patients with bilateral IOM.[37]

One of our FAMMM kindreds has been followed for at least two decades. CMM is present in three generations — III, IV, and V (see Figure 6, Part A). AN have been identified in three generations — IV, V, and VI — with some members having both CMM and AN (IV-8, V-5,V-6, and V-7). Two additional members of the pedigree (see Figure 6, Part A, III-3, IV-1) are decreased and had verified CMM (see Table 6). Within this section of the pedigree there were four members who had systemic cancer, but only two were examined

TABLE 5
Tumor Registry of Dutch Kindred

Patient	Sex	Age @ Ca onset	Age @ death	Cancer Dx	Ca site	Verif.	Clin. DN	Histol. DN
II-2	M	45	49	CMM	Sk	PR		
II-7	M	?	84	CMM	Sk	PR	+	+
				Sq Cell	Lx	PR		
II-10	F	60		AC	Br	PR		
		65	66	CMM	Sk	PR		
II-11	F	66		Ca	Br	PR		
		69	75	CMM	Sk	PR	−	
III-1	M	48	48	CMM	Sk	PR		
III-4	M	46	48	Ca	Lu	PR		
III-8	M	53		CMM	Sk	PR	+	+
		55		CMM	Sk	PR		
		57		IOM	R eye	PR		
		58	58	IOM	L eye	PR		
III-9	M						+	
III-10	F	51	51	CMM	Sk	PR		
III-12	F	58	59	CMM	Sk	PR	−	
IV-4	F						−	
IV-5	F	28		CMM	Sk	PR	+	+
IV-6	F						+	+
IV-7	M						−	−
IV-8	M						+	
IV-9	F	22		CMM	Sk	PR	−	
IV-10	M						+	

Note: Ca = cancer; CMM = cutaneous malignant melanoma; Sq Cell = squamous cell; AC = anaplastic carcinoma; IOM = intraocular melanoma; DN = dysplastic nevi; PR = pathology report; Sk = skin; Lx = larynx; Lu = lung; Br = breast; + = examined, FAMMM nevi; − = examined, normal nevi.

for AN. One of these was at 50% risk (IV-10) and had normal moles and no AN, but did have Hodgkin's disease. Another member at 25% risk had classical AN and cervical carcinoma *in situ*. One of the deceased members who had CMM (III-3) had four children. Only one of her four progeny had classical AN on cutaneous examination. To date, we have examined the skin of 12 members of the extended pedigree plotted in Part B (see Figure 6). Only two members of that extended pedigree had AN clinically, which is not adequate to establish whether this part of the pedigree has the FAMMM genotype. Examination of additional family members is necessary to firmly establish the FAMMM genotype in the extended Part B of Figure 6 of the Nebraska kindred.

Finally, these patients with multiple primary CMMs show unusual increased survival. For example, one patient (our original proband) over 2 decades had 13 separate primary CMMs, of which two were nodular Clark's IV lesions.[7,47]

Collectively, these clinical/pathological/genetic findings in our four FAMMM kindreds indicate a possibly unique host factor mechanism in the natural history of cancer expression. These observations cover a panorama ranging from cancer resistance to precocious expression of cancer, including variable penetrance and expressivity of the phenotype by a single dominant gene with high penetrance. This is pertinent since clinical evaluation of our patients showed clear evidence of variable expressivity of the phenotype, thereby posing diagnostic difficulty, particularly when an isolated case is encountered showing incomplete expression of the FAMMM phenotype. The important lesson from these observations is that we must not view the patient in isolation but rather in the broader context of his genotypic status. The genotypic status can only be evaluated by a detailed pedigree analysis.

TABLE 6
Tumor Registry of North P Kindred (Parts A & B)

Patient	Sex	Age @ Ca onset	Age @ death	Cancer Dx	Ca site	Verif.	Clin. DN	Histol. DN
				1299-A				
III-3	F	54	61	CMM	Sk	PR		
III-5	M	53		CMM	Sk	PR		
		62	62	Sq Cell	Lu	PR		
III-6	F						–	–
III-7	M	52	52	Sq Cell	Lu	PR		
IV-1	F	57	60	CMM	Sk	PR	–	–
IV-3	F						+	–
IV-5	M	51		Astro	Bra	PR		
IV-8	F	23		CMM	Sk	PR	+	+
IV-10	M	29		Hodg	Lym	PR	–	–
V-5	F	18		CMM	Sk	PR	+	+
		22		CMM	Sk	PR		
		23		CMM × 2	Sk	PR		
		32		CMM	Sk			
V-6	M	23		CMM	Sk	PR	+	–
V-7	M	33		CMM × 2	Sk	PR	+	+
V-8	F	30		CIS	Cx	PR	+	–
V-9	F						–	
V-10	M						–	
V-11	M						–	
V-13	M						–	
V-15	M						–	
V-16	M						–	
VI-1	M						+	
VI-2	M						+	
				1229-B				
II-2	M	50	52	Ca	St	DC		
II-7	M		73	Ca	Lu	DC		
II-8	F	59	61	Lym sarc	Lym	DC		
III-8	M	88		Adeno	Co			
III-10	M		87	Ca	Pro	DC		
III-15	F	50		Cystaden	Ov	MR		
		55	57	Ca	Panc	MR		
III-16	F			Ca	St	FR		
III-18	M	61		Ca	Pro	PR	–	
IV-14	F						–	
IV-22	M			Ca	CSU	FR		
V-20	F	39	41	Ca	Br	PR		
V-22	M						+	
V-24	M						+	

Note: Adeno = adenocarcinoma; Astro = astocytoma; Br = breast; Ca = cancer; CIS = carcinoma *in situ*; CMM = cutaneous malignant melanoma; Co = colon; CSU = cancer site unknown; Cystadeno = cystadenocarcinoma; Cx = cervix; DC = death certificate; DN = dysplastic nevi; FR = family report; Hodg = Hodgkin's disease; Lu = lung; Lym = lymphoma; Lym Sarc = lymphosarcoma; MR = medical record; Ov = ovary; Panc = pancreas; PR = pathology report; Pro = prostate; Sk = skin; Sq cell = squamous cell; St = stomach; + = examined, FAMMM nevi; – = examined, normal nevi.

X. POLYGENIC INHERITANCE AND THE FAMMM

Traupe et al.[56] have argued that a polygenic model, as opposed to autosomal dominant inheritance, may provide a better explanation for the genetics of the FAMMM syndrome. This supposition has been based on an apparent lack of genetic equilibrium between newly arising and eliminated mutations which these investigators believe is not compatible with the postulated autosomal dominantly inherited mechanism for the FAMMM.

Clearly, we cannot exclude a polygenic inheritance model for certain occurrences of the FAMMM syndrome or for so-called sporadic occurrences of either dysplastic nevi or the syndrome per se. However, we believe that there are many serious problems which Traupe et al.[56] failed to address when they compiled their mutation rate estimates for the FAMMM. Specifically, in spite of more than a decade of interest in the FAMMM, we are aware of countless situations wherein patients have been considered to be sporadic occurrences of the disorder when, in fact, a sufficiently detailed history had not been obtained. Our own evaluation of many of these so-called sporadic examples of the FAMMM, following in-depth family studies, has shown a pattern of transmission consonant with an autosomal dominantly inherited factor. Another problem pertains to the significance of occasional AN vs. a more prolific form which would be readily recognized by most clinicians as representing the FAMMM phenotype. If the clinician has a patient with occasional or isolated AN and failed to examine the skin of the patient's primary and secondary relatives, he may consider the case as a sporadic. On the other hand, we take the position based on our clinical experience that isolated or only occasional AN may represent an extreme end of the continuum of the FAMMM due to variable expressivity of the AN phenotype.

These points are raised in that they could seriously distort estimates of not only the frequency of the FAMMM genotype, but also, the expression of the trait within families. Finally, we have called attention to the possibility of heterogeneity in the FAMMM per se so that there may well be more than one allelic FAMMM syndrome(s) (see Figure 1).

In conclusion, we continue to believe that an autosomal dominant mode of genetic transmission is the best model for explaining its genetic etiology, as evidenced by our formal segregation analysis[53] and the recognition of vertical transmission within our extended pedigrees.

XI. EXTRA-MELANOTIC CANCER AND THE FAMMM

The issue of whether or not certain extra-melanotic cancers are integral to the FAMMM has been controversial. We believe that much of this controversy can be explained on the basis of the methodological approaches to this problem which have been employed in certain of these studies. Specifically, there has been a failure by some of our colleagues to perform meticulous documentation of cancer of *all* anatomic sites within *extended* kindreds. In addition, the likelihood of tumor heterogeneity within the FAMMM has not been given serious consideration by these researchers.

Bergman et al.[57] investigated cancer of *all* anatomic sites in nine FAMMM kindreds which were ascertained in a pigmented lesions clinic in the Netherlands. A significant excess of systemic cancer (particularly involving the gastrointestinal tract) was observed in three of these nine families. The remaining families showed normal expectations of cancer among FAMMM gene carriers and their first degree relatives based on Dutch incidence data. Of the 18 gastrointestinal tract cancers, 9 involved the pancreas, while none were colorectal cancer. This was compared with Dutch incidence data in which half of the gastrointestinal tract cancers were of the colorectum, while approximately 10% involved the pancreas. All of the pancreatic cancers were adenocarcinomas. The fact that three of these nine families showed a marked excess of systemic cancer, while the remaining families showed normal numbers of cancer among those with the FAMMM genotype and their first degree relatives, indicated significant heterogeneity to exist among these families.

In contrast, studies of the FAMMM syndrome which claim to have demonstrated a negative history for systemic cancer excess have been deficient in their verification methodology. Kopf et al.[58] reported no evidence for systemic cancer in patients with familial malignant melanoma. An analysis of the data showed the methodology to have been based on interview, physical examination, and questionnaire, which was restricted to the proband and his recall of family history. This study did not involve contacting *other* members of the family; therefore, it was *not* an in-depth genetic study and dose not contribute to the understanding of hereditary malignant melanoma, and its natural history, inclusive of systemic cancer association. Lynch et al.[59] have shown in the past that restrictive genetic investigations which rely on limited recall of the proband give misleading data with respect to cancer occurrences in the kindred.

Greene et al.[60] performed a prospective study of 14 kindreds at the NIH with hereditary CMM and the dysplastic nevus syndrome. They concluded that "no significant excess of nonmelanoma cancers was documented, suggesting that hereditary cutaneous malignant melanoma/dysplastic nevus syndrome are not pleiotropic for other tumor types." These conclusions were based on a negative finding which is weak in its statistical power, and both restrictive and biased in its patient selection. The study covers an approximate 5-year period and is not adequate for the development of the phenotypic expression of systemic cancer which in hereditary cancer syndromes requires several generations for development of characteristic patterns. If one calculates the expression of systemic cancer with the use of only defined gene carriers (those with dysplastic nevi and/or malignant melanoma), their data show that there is a significant increase in the occurrence of gastrointestinal cancer ($p < 0.05$). Since these numbers were small, the authors considered them to be insufficient to support the hypothesis of an excess of nonmelanotic cancer in the dysplastic nevus syndrome. It would be important to know in this study if the cancers were limited to only a few kindreds rather than all 14 kindreds. This question has been asked, but not answered. If it were restricted to a few kindred, it would verify the concept of heterogeneity which appears to be common in cancer-associated genodermatoses, thus increasing the significance of the cancer finding because of the smaller cohort size of the gene carriers.

XII. CYTOGENETIC AND GENE LINKAGE STUDIES AND THE FAMMM

Appropriately, research has focused on chromosomal localization of the gene for DNS. Noteworthy was the report by Bale et al.[61] which involved the study of 99 relatives and 26 spouses in six families who were predisposed to melanoma. Thirty-four of these individuals had CMM, while 31 of these 34 showed histologic confirmation of DN. Twenty-four relatives showed DN alone. These findings indicated that the deleterious gene was on the distal part of the short arm of chromosome 1 (1p36) in a region between an anonymous DNA marker (D1S47) and the gene locus for pronatrodilatin (PND). The probe for D1S47 and PND showed lod scores of 3.62 and 3.09, respectively. The authors concluded that the odds were greater than 260,000:1 in support of linkage at this location.

However, van Haeringen et al.[63] performed linkage studies in six large Dutch DNS families. These investigators failed to find support for linkage between the loci for DNS and the rhesus blood group on chromosome 1. They concluded that "...data from additional markers (DNF15S1, D1Z2, FUCA1, D1S17, D1S57, and PGM1) make it possible to exclude the DNS gene from the short arm of chromosome 1 in these Dutch families."

In collaboration with Leppert and White, we have also excluded linkage on the short arm of chromosome 1 in the investigation of two extended FAMMM kindreds. These findings will be the subject of a future report.

An explanation for these discrepant findings remains elusive. It is possible that heterogeneity among the American[61] and the Dutch[62] HDNS kindreds could have contributed to some of these discrepancies. Variable expressivity and penetrance of the FAMMM gene must also be considered. In addition, there is an absence of any well-defined and accepted criteria for the minimal expression needed for FAMMM's diagnosis in individual patients. Specifically, this is evidenced by the fact that a genotypically affected patient may have a complete absence of FAMMM moles,[4] and yet express CMM. On the other hand, a patient may have neither DN, CMM, or other systemic cancer, but be an obligate gene carrier by virtue of his or her position within the pedigree.[48]

Jaspers et al.[62] performed cytogenetic investigations on 25 individuals who were members of six DNS kindreds. Comparison was made among patients with DNS without a history of melanoma and their clinically normal relatives, as well as unrelated normal controls. These investigators indicated that normal frequencies of hyperdiploidy and spontaneous sister chromatid exchanges (SCE) in fibroblasts from these individuals were present. Karyotypic studies were conducted on the relatives from one of these kindreds. Of interest was the finding that "...DNS had a normal constitutional karyotype. In lymphocytes or fibroblasts from five patients, however, increased frequencies of cells with random chromosomal rearrangements were observed. These abnormalities, mainly translocations and inversions, were not found in two of the patients' spouses and in six clinically normal relatives. In the fibroblast cultures, considerable clonal selection of cytogenetically abnormal cells occurred."

In collaboration with Sandberg, we have studied cytogenetics from cultured lymphocytes, skin, and AN from two extended FAMMM kindreds. Findings showed significant chromosomal breakage and nonrandom translocations. These abnormalities were observed primarily in AN and normal skin fibroblasts.[64] It will now be important to verify our cytogenetic findings in other well-documented FAMMM kindreds. It will be equally important to determine whether these cytogenetic findings might be capable of predicting differences in phenotypic expression of DN, CMM, and systemic cancer among FAMMM patients/families. This cytogenetic marker(s) should also be helpful in identifying individuals who are presumptive obligate gene carriers but who otherwise have not expressed any stigmata of the FAMMM phenotype. Its value will also extend to the identification of persons who have subtle phenotypic findings but who clinically may be considered either equivocal or unaffected. It will be imperative to follow such patients in order to determine whether CMM and cancers of extra-melanotic sites occur in association with these cytogenetic aberrations. Finally, the cytogenetic marker(s) should also be evaluated in the following settings: (1) patients with sporadic atypical nevi and/or CMM and (2) kindreds with familial melanoma in the *absence* of FAMMM phenotypic features.

XIII. DISCUSSION

Our experience in the evaluation of thousands of hereditary cancer-prone families of all varieties, inclusive of melanoma, has indicated to us that the identification of hereditary forms of CMM, as well as IOM, may be complicated by a myriad of confounding variables. Elucidation of these problems may also be hampered by the limited knowledge about genetics among these at risk patients' primary physicians. It would appear secure that the FAMMM is a dominantly inherited cancer-associated genodermatosis. What is not clear is the question of modifying genes that will affect the phenotypic expression as seen in the fish melanoma model that has been investigated by Anders in Germany. It may well be that there is parallelism present in hereditary melanoma in fish and man. We can learn much about human melanoma genetics through the investigation of this disease in fish, as pioneered by Anders.

Knowledge of the spectrum of cutaneous phenotypic traits that characterize hereditary CMM syndromes is crucial. However, variations in clinical expression of phenotype are extant and thereby require in depth clinical and genetic analysis of the patients and their families. This subject is discussed by Fusaro and Lynch in the chapter dealing with phenotypic variation in the FAMMM.

The study of our schematic that portrays our unifying etiologic hypothesis for MM mandates that one always consider environmental interaction within the context of the basic human gene pool. Clearly, environmental perturbations are influenced by the macromilieu of chemical, physical (particularly sunlight), and nutritional factors, and the micromilieu of endogenous biological agents, such as oncogenes, tumor suppressor genes, and viruses, all of which act in concert to modify the basic genetic expression of the human disease.[7]

It is clear that the FAMMM syndrome is now recognized as a disorder which constitutes a significant fraction of the overall malignant melanoma burden. The public health significance of the problem is immense given the fact that CMM is reaching veritably epidemic proportions in those sun belt areas of the world inhabited by large numbers of Caucasians. It is therefore appropriate to ask, "Will the statistical fraction of the FAMMM increase or decrease in proportion to the increasing incidence of CMM in these high risk geographic regions?" This question is important since it has a bearing on whether or not solar radiation is unmasking a genetic susceptibility to CMM which, in a non-sun belt area and/or among individuals who are employing protection from the sun's rays, through use of clothing, sun screens, or less leisure activity in the sun, have a *lesser* incidence of phenotype (CMM) expression. Until pharmacologic and/or genetic engineering products/procedures [are available?], which can prevent the genetic expression of phenotype — melanoma — we must adapt the single most important, immediate, preventive medical care that can be adapted with little expense; that is, the return to limited sunlight exposure.

We have raised many additional questions throughout the course of this chapter. For example, we wonder whether the risk for CMM is the same in all FAMMM kindreds or whether there may be marked heterogeneity with respect to the occurrence of CMM within and between FAMMM kindreds. We also wonder about the percentage of AN in the general population, with particular attention to how many individuals with AN may, in fact, have the FAMMM syndrome. There have been estimates that perhaps 5 to 9% of the Caucasian population around the world have atypical moles (DN).

A dilemma pertains to so-called "sporadic" occurrences of atypical moles vs. their classical presentation in the autosomal dominantly inherited setting of an extended FAMMM kindred. Clearly, as outlined in the chapter on cutaneous manifestations, there are limitations which must be imposed upon the term sporadic as it is an operational or investigative term. It is important to note, however, that the ability to distinguish sporadic from genetic, in the case of the FAMMM, will be resolved once a biomarker of acceptable sensitivity and specificity to the FAMMM genotype becomes available.

Another question pertains to the presence or absence of non-melanoma cancer occurrences in the FAMMM. This concern may relate to our postulated view that the FAMMM is heterogeneous and that not only the mentioned frequency of melanoma may vary, but also the incidence of systemic forms of cancer may show variability within and between FAMMM kindreds.

These questions, and many others which could readily be generated, will undoubtedly be answered through multidisciplined collaborative investigations of large numbers of FAMMM kindreds. Needed will be multigenerational studies wherein meticulous care is given to the distribution and documentation of cancer of *all* anatomic sites in concert with the numerous facets of the natural history and cutaneous phenotype of the FAMMM.

When one considers the history of science, it should not be surprising that newly discovered diseases and/or the increasing incidence of a particular disorder will serve as a stimulus for research on its genetic epidemiology. The AIDS epidemic is a clear-cut example of this phenomenon. Economic factors (available funding), ease, and efficiency of available research tools, as well as new insights into the etiology of the disorder also serve to influence priority to, and the framing of, specific research goals and objectives. Collectively, these factors have clearly fashioned the genetic epidemiology of specific forms of CMM. Needed in this research is the recognition that neither environmental nor genetic factors operate in a vacuum. Rather, it is an understanding of their interaction which will provide crucial clues to etiology in the multifaceted process of carcinogenesis in MM.

REFERENCES

1. **Koh, H. K. and Rogers, G. S.,** Malignant melanoma: early detection and treatment, in *Primary Care,* Vol. 16, Pariser, R. J., Ed., W. B. Saunders, Philadelphia, 1989, sect. 3.
2. **Roser, M., Bohm, A., Oldigs, M., Weichenthal, M., Reimers, U., Schmidt-Preuss, U., Breitbart, E. W., and Rudiger, H. W.,** Ultraviolet-induced formation of micronuclei and sister chromatid exchange in cultured fibroblasts of patients with cutaneous malignant melanoma, *Cancer Genet. Cytogenet.,* 41, 129, 1989.
3. **Lynch, H. T. and Fusaro, R. M.,** Hereditary malignant melanoma: a unifying etiologic hypothesis, *Cancer Genet. Cytogenet.* 20, 301, 1986.
4. **Lynch, H. T., Fusaro, R. M., Danes, B. S., Lynch, J. F., and Kimberling, W. J.,** A review of hereditary malignant melanoma, including biomarkers in the FAMMM, *Cancer Genet. Cytogenet.,* 8, 325, 1983.
5. **Mosher, D. B., Fitzpatrick, T. B., Ortonne, J. P., and Hori, Y.,** Disorders of pigmentation, in *Dermatology in General Medicine,* 3rd ed., Fitzpatrick, T. B., Eisen, A. S., Wolff, K., Freedberg, I. M., and Austen, K. F., Eds., McGraw-Hill, New York, 1987, 803.
6. **Schulze, K. E., Rapini, R. P., and Duvic, M.,** Malignant melanoma in oculocutaneous albinism, *Arch. Dermatol.,* 125, 1583, 1989.
7. **Lynch, H. T. and Fusaro, R. M.,** *Cancer-Associated Genodermatoses,* Van Nostrand Reinhold, New York, 1982.
8. **Cleaver, J. E.,** Defective repair replication of DNA in xeroderma pigmentosum, *Nature (London),* 218, 652, 1968.
9. **Johnson, R. T., Elliott, G. C., Squires, S., and Joysey, V. C.,** Lack of complementation between xeroderma pigmentosum complementation groups D and H, *Hum. Genet.,* 81, 203, 1989.
10. **Bootsma, D., Keijzer, W., Jung, E. G., and Bohnert, E.,** Xeroderma pigmentosum complementation group XP-I withdrawn, *Mutat. Res.,* 218, 149, 1989.
11. **Kraemer, K. H.,** Xeroderma pigmentosum, in *Clinical Dermatology,* Demis, D. J., Dobson, R. L. and McGuire, J., Eds., Harper & Row, New York, 1980, unit 19-7.
12. **Lynch, H. T., Frichot, B. C., Fisher, J., et al.,** Spontaneous regression of metastatic malignant melanoma in two sibs with xeroderma pigmentation, *J. Med. Genet.,* 15, 357, 1978.
13. **Nathanson, L.,** Spontaneous regression of malignant melanoma: a review of the literature on incidence, clinical features, and possible mechanisms, *Natl. Cancer Inst. Monog.,* 44, 57, 1976.
14. **Lynch, H. T., Fusaro, R. M., and Johnson, J. A.,** Xeroderma pigmentosum — complementation group C and malignant melanoma, *Arch. Dermatol.,* 120, 175, 1984.
15. **Robbins, J. H., Kraemer, K. H., Lutzner, M. A., et al.,** Xeroderma pigmentosum: an inherited disease with sun sensitivity, multiple cutaneous neoplasms, and abnormal DNA repair, *Ann. Intern. Med.,* 80, 221, 1974.
16. **Greely, P. W., Middleton, A. G., and Curtin, J. W.,** Incidence of malignancy in giant pigmented nevi, *Plast. Reconstr. Surg.,* 36, 26, 1965.
17. **Kaplan, E. N.,** The risk of malignancy in large congenital nevi, *Plast. Reconstr. Surg.,* 53, 421, 1974.
18. **Lewis, M. G.,** Melanoma and pigmentation of the leptomeninges in Ugandan Africans, *J. Clin. Pathol.,* 22, 183, 1969.
19. **Lorentzen, M., et al.,** Incidence of malignant transformation in giant pigmented nevi, *Scand. J. Plast. Reconstr. Surg.,* 11, 163, 1977.
20. **Pers, M.,** Naevus pigmentosus giganticus, *Ugeskr Laeg.,* 125, 613, 1963.
21. **Reed, W. B., et al.,** Giant pigmented nevi, melanoma, and leptomeningeal melanocytosis, *Arch. Dermatol.* 91, 100, 1965.
22. **Russell, J. L. and Reyes, R. G.,** Giant pigmented nevi, *JAMA,* 171, 2083, 1959.

23. **Goodman, R. M., et al.**, Genetic considerations in giant pigmented hairy nevus, *Br. J. Dermatol.* 85, 100, 1971.
24. **Voigtlander, V. and Jung, E. E.**, Giant pigmented hairy nevus in two siblings, *Humangenetik,* 24, 79, 1974.
25. **Traboulsi, E. I., Zimmerman, L. E., and Manz, H. J.**, Cutaneous malignant melanoma in survivors of heritable retinoblastoma, *Arch. Ophthalmol.,* 106, 1059, 1988.
26. **Strong, L. C., Herson, J., Haas, C., Elder, K., Chakraborty, R., Weiss, K. M., and Majunder, P.**, Cancer mortality in relatives of retinoblastoma patients, *JNCI,* 73, 303, 1984.
27. **Hogan, M. J. and Zimmerman, L. E.**, *Ophthalmic Pathology: An Atlas and Textbook,* 2nd ed., W. B. Saunders, Philadelphia, 1962, 413.
28. **Allen, J. C. and Jaeschke, U. H.**, Recurrence of malignant melanoma in an orbit after 28 years, *Arch. Ophthalmol.,* 79, 1966.
29. **Bowen, S. F., Brady, H., and Jones, V. L.**, Malignant melanoma of the eye occurring in two successive generations, *Arch. Ophthalmol.,* 71, 805, 1964.
30. **Davenport, R. C.**, A family history of choroidal sarcoma, *Br. J. Ophthalmol.,* 11, 443, 1927.
31. **Gutmann, G.**, Casuistischer Beitrag zur Lehre von de Geschwulsten des Augapfels, *Arch. Augenheilkunde,* 31, 158, 1895.
32. **Parsons, J. H.**, *The Pathology of the Eye — Histology,* Part II, Vol. 2, G. P. Putnam's Sons, New York, 1095, 496.
33. **Pfingst, A. O. and Graves, S.**, Melanosarcoma of choroid occurring in brothers, *Arch. Ophthalmol.,* 50, 431, 1921.
34. **Silcock, A. Q.**, Hereditary sarcoma of eyeball in three generations, *Br. Med. J.,* 1, 1079, 1892.
35. **Waardenburg, P. J.**, Melanosarcoma of eye in various members of the same family with report of case, *Ned. Geneesk.,* 84, 4718, 1940.
36. **Lynch, H. T., Fusaro, R. M., Pester, J., Oosterhuis, J. A., Went, L. N., Rumke, P., Neering, H., and Lynch, J. F.**, Tumor spectrum in the FAMMM syndrome, *Br. J. Cancer,* 44, 553, 1981.
37. **Oosterhuis, J. A., Went, L. N., and Lynch, H. T.**, Primary choroidal and cutaneous melanomas, bilateral choroidal melanomas, and familial occurrence of melanomas, *Br. J. Ophthalmol.,* 66, 230, 1982.
38. **Lynch, H. T., Anderson, D. E., and Krush, A. J.**, Heredity and intraocular malignant melanoma — study of two families and review of 45 cases, *Cancer,* 21, 119, 1968.
39. Consensus conference: precursors to malignant melanoma, *JAMA,* 251, 1864, 1984.
40. **Norris, W.**, A case of fungoid disease, *Edin. Med. Surg. J.,* 16, 562, 1820.
41. **Cawley, E. P.**, Genetic aspects of malignant melanoma, *Arch. Dermatol., Syphilol.,* 65, 440, 1952.
42. **Lynch, H. T., Frichot, B. C., and Lynch, J. F.**, Familial atypical multiple mole melanoma syndrome, *J. Med. Genet.,* 15, 352, 1978.
43. **Clark, W. H., Reimer, R. R., Greene, M., Ainsworth, A. M., and Mastrangelo, M. J.**, Origin of familial malignant melanoma from heritable melanocytic lesions: the B-K mole syndrome, *Arch. Dermatol.,* 114, 732, 1978.
44. **Elder, D. E., Goldman, L. I., Goldman, S. C., Greene, M. H., and Clark, W. H.**, Dysplastic nevus syndrome: a phenotypic association of sporadic cutaneous melanoma, *Cancer,* 46, 1787, 1980.
45. **Bondi, E. E., Clark, W. H., Elder, D., Guerry, D., and Greene, M. H.**, Topical chemotherapy of dysplastic melanocytic nevi with 5% fluorouracil, *Arch. Dermatol.,* 117, 89, 1981.
46. **Kopf, A. W., Hellman, L. J., Rogers, G. S., Gross, D. F., Rigel, D. S., Friedman, R. J., Levenstein, M., Brown, J., Golomb, F. M., Roses, D. F., Gumport, S. L., and Mintzis, M. M.**, Familial malignant melanoma, *JAMA,* 256, 1915, 1986.
47. **Lynch, H. T., and Krush, A. J.**, Heredity and malignant melanoma: implications for cancer detection, *Can. Med. Assoc. J.,* 99, 17, 1968.
48. **Lynch, H. T., Fusaro, R. M., Pester, J., and Lynch, J.**, Familial atypical multiple mole melanoma (FAMMM) syndrome: genetic heterogeneity and malignant melanoma, *Br. J. Cancer,* 42, 58, 1980.
49. **Lynch, H. T., Fusaro, R. M., Pester, J., Albano, W. A., and Lynch, J. F.**, Phenotypic variation in the familial atypical multiple mole melanoma syndrome (FAMMM), *J. Med. Genet.,* 20, 25, 1983a.
50. **Lynch, H. T., Fusaro, R. M., Kimberling, W. J., and Lynch, J. F.**, The cutaneous evolution of nevi in a patient with familial atypical multiple mole melanoma syndrome, *Ped. Dermatol.,* 2, 289, 1985.
51. **Frichot, B. C., Lynch, H. T., Guirgis, H. A., Harris, R. E., and Lynch, J. F.**, A new cutaneous phenotype in familial malignant melanoma, *Lancet,* 1,864, 1977.
52. **Lynch, H. T., Frichot, B. C., Lynch, P. M., Lynch, J., and Guirgis, H. A.**, Family studies of malignant melanoma and associated cancer, *SGO,* 141, 517, 1975.
53. **Lynch, H. T., Fusaro, R. M., Kimberling, W. J., and Lynch, J. F.**, Familial atypical multiple mole melanoma (FAMMM) syndrome: segregation analysis, *J. Med. Genet.,* 20, 342, 1983a.
54. **Cutler, S. J. and Young, J. L.**, The Third National Cancer Survey: Incidence Data, *Natl. Cancer Inst. Monog.,* 41, 1975.

55. **Bellet, R. E., Shields, J. A., Soll, D. B., and Bernardino, E. A.,** Primary choroidal and cutaneous melanomas occurring in a patient with the B-K mole syndrome phenotype, *Am. J. Ophthalmol.*, 89, 567, 1980.
56. **Traupe, H., Macher, E., Hamm, H., and Happle, R.,** Mutation rate estimates are not compatible with autosomal dominant inheritance of the dysplastic nevus "syndrome", *Am. J. Hum. Genet.*, 32, 155, 1989.
57. **Bergman, W., Watson, P., deJong, J., Lynch, H. T., and Fusaro, R. M.,** Systemic cancer and the FAMMM syndrome, *Br. J. Cancer,* 61, 932, 1990.
58. **Kopf, A. W., Friedman, R. J., and Rigesl, D. S.,** Atypical mole syndrome, *JAAD,* 22, 117, 1990.
59. **Lynch, H. T., Follett, K. L., Lynch, P. M., Albano, W. A., Mailliard, J. A., and Pierson, R. L.,** Family history in an oncology clinic: implications for cancer genetics, *JAMA,* 242, 1268, 1979.
60. **Greene, M. H., Tucker, M. A., Clark, W. H., Kraemer, K. H., Elder, D. E., and Fraser, M. C.,** Hereditary melanoma and the dysplastic nevus syndrome: the risk of cancers other than melanoma, *JAAD,* 16, 792, 1987.
61. **Bale, S. J., Dracopoli, N. C., Tucker, M. A., Clark, W. H., Fraser, M. C., Stanger, B. Z., Green, P., Donis-Keller, H., Housman, D. E., and Greene, M. H.,** Mapping the gene for hereditary cutaneous malignant melanoma-dysplastic nevus to chromosome 1p, *N. Engl. J. Med.*, 320, 1367, 1989.
62. **Jaspers, N. G. J., Roza-deJongh, E. J. M., Donselaar, I. G., vanVelzen-Tillemans, J. T. M., vanHemel, J. O., Rumke, P., and vanderKamp, A. W. M.,** Sister chromatid exchanges, hyperdiploidy, and chromosomal rearrangements studied in cells from melanoma-prone individuals belonging to families with the dysplastic nevus syndrome, *Cancer Genet. Cytogenet.*, 24, 33, 1987.
63. **van Haeringen, A., Bergman, W., Nelen, M. R., van der Koou-Meijs, E., Hendrikse, I., Wijnen, J. T., Meera Khan, P., Klasen, E. C., and Frants, R. R.,** Exclusion of the dysplastic nevus syndrome (DNS) locus from the short arm of chromosome 1 by linkage studies in Dutch families, *Genomics,* 5, 61, 1989.
64. **Lynch, H. T. et al.,** in preparation.

Chapter 2

THE CUTANEOUS MANIFESTATIONS OF THE FAMILIAL ATYPICAL MULTIPLE MOLE MELANOMA (FAMMM) SYNDROME

Ramon M. Fusaro and Henry T. Lynch

TABLE OF CONTENTS

I. INTRODUCTION

The cutaneous manifestations of the familial atypical multiple mole melanoma (FAMMM) syndrome (hereditary dysplastic nevus syndrome — HDNS) have only been recognized since the middle of the 1970s by two different independent research groups.[1,2] This disorder has been established by several investigative teams[1-5] to be an autosomal dominantly inherited trait with incomplete penetrance, variable expressivity of phenotype, and heterogeneity of the genotype. The characteristic cutaneous findings in members of kindreds with the classical presentation of this disorder are (1) the occurrence of increased incidence of cutaneous malignant melanoma (CMM); (2) the members of the kindred can have an increased number of total body nevi with counts greater than normal; and (3) the presence of multiple large atypical nevi which are usually clinically distinguishable from normal nevi when greater than 4 mm in diameter. This disorder has gone through the usual evolution of new discoveries; that is, there is sudden enlightenment followed by an increasing insecurity of understanding of the pathogenesis, as new information accrues.

II. HISTORICAL PERSPECTIVE

Norris in 1820 reported the first description of a family with a hereditary form of CMM (a FAMMM kindred?).[6] His discovery lay dormant for well over a century before Cawley, a dermatologist, in 1952 described a contemporary family with hereditary malignant melanoma in a father and two of his three children; however, no clear clinical notation was made of the classic cutaneous phenotypes of the FAMMM.[7] It may well be that the family reported by Cawley was not a FAMMM syndrome. Prior to the identification of the FAMMM kindreds by Lynch et al.,[1] this research group from Creighton University described one of these FAMMM families in 1968 as it appeared to have hereditary CMM in the kindred.[8] The cutaneous phenotypes were not recognized as distinctive at that time. This cancer associated genodermatosis has obviously been present in the Caucasian population for many millennia. It has been described in Europe, the U.S., and Australia but it also has been observed in Asia in non-Caucasians.

Why wasn't this condition recognized before 1977? Dermatologists who have been practicing many years will relate that, in retrospect, they can remember having seen patients with CMM and lots of moles with some of them being atypical nevi. There are probably multiple reasons that the FAMMM syndrome was only recently discovered, but the most obvious is that our concepts of hereditary cancer and its prevalence have changed from a very rare condition to the conservative possibility of accounting for at least 10% or more of today's overall cancer burden.[9] Clearly, a significant impediment to knowledge about the FAMMM syndrome is the fact that dermatologists and oncologists did not take adequate genetic histories to establish an hereditary concept. Recognition of the observations that in FAMMM families some members of the kindred had malignant melanoma, total body count of moles almost too numerous to count, and many atypical nevi, were therefore not possible. To further obfuscate the recognition of the FAMMM syndrome is the fact that patients in the vast majority of instances do not know accurately the medical history of their immediate family (first degree relatives) let alone about their second degree relatives.[10] In addition, the concept of occurrence of nevi, melanoma, congenital nevi, and risk factors for malignant degeneration of melanocytic nevi has only evolved in a meaningful manner within the last two decades, thereby enabling us to better understand the pathogenesis of malignant melanoma.

TABLE 1
Clinical and Temporal Findings of the Cutaneous FAMMM Phenotypes

Characteristics[a]	Clinical expression
Number of total nevi (both atypical [AN] and normal nevi) {1,3}	Greater than normal count: often 50 to 100 or more with lesions of all sizes and shapes (heterogeneous); unknown: percentage of normal vs. AN; the lower limits of number have not been defined
Size of AN {1,2,3,4}	Size from 4—5 mm or greater, the lower limits of size recognition unknown
Border of AN {1,3,4}	Serpiginous or irregular with color leakage (fading) into the periphery but the border can be sharp and oval or round with no pigment fading at periphery
Color of AN {1,2,3,4}	Variegate: red, tan, brown, and almost black; single lesions occasionally can be only one color
Contour of AN {3,4}	Usually macular but can be raised centrally with the surface occasionally mammillated (fine cobblestones)
Anatomic location of AN {1,2,3,4}	The trunk prominently and the proximal extremities next, but scalp in both sexes and legs in females; the face, sole, and palms are invariably spared
Age of recognition of AN {2}	Puberty, description of AN in children is limited but AN (>4 mm) have been reported in children
Rate of change and time span of presence {2}	Usually nevi start appearing early in the first decade of life with number greater than normal; new nevi continue to appear into the fourth and fifth decades of life; the AN can especially increase in size and shape and change color; all nevi regress in the sixth through the eighth decade of life
Normal nevi in FAMMM {1}	Present but in greater number than normal; however, the extent and definition has not been determined
Malignant melanoma {4}	Presence of CMM with other phenotypes of AN and/or increased total mole count but CMM can be present in the absence of any nevi, CMMs appear after puberty, not all FAMMM kindreds develop CMM in their members

[a] The number of the color plates which illustrate these morphological characteristics are listed as arabic numbers enclosed in braces {#} under the column — Characteristics.

III. CUTANEOUS MORPHOLOGY AND TEMPORAL RELATIONSHIPS

To the informed dermatologist, the classic florid cutaneous expressions of the FAMMM syndrome are easily recognized at a glance without the slightest hesitation. Because of the variable expressivity, incomplete penetrance of the trait and the heterogeneity of the genotype, the precise definition of the morphological spectrum of expression of the cutaneous lesions are extremely more complex than originally conceived. The minimal expression of all the clinical characteristics has not been defined or studied in an orderly manner that would encompass the genetic nature of the disorder. The known and unknown cutaneous phenotypic findings of patients with the FAMMM syndrome are summarized in Table 1.*

IV. VARIABLE EXPRESSIVITY OF THE FAMMM PHENOTYPES

As the child with the FAMMM phenotype grows older, the clinical changes in the phenotype of the atypical nevi can be described with the ABCDE designation: (A) the lesions become increasingly asymmetrical; (B) the border becomes more serpiginous and notched; (C) the color changes become more variable and variegated; (D) the diameter approaches 4

* Plates 1 to 4 appear following page 30.

to 5 mm and greater; and (E) the macular lesions can develop a central elevation or the surface becomes mammillated (fine cobblestones). If all these clinical characteristics are exaggerated further to their extremes then the ABCDE become the characteristics of the early clinical morphology of CMM. At this end of the clinical spectrum, the clinical separation of the florid atypical nevus and early CMM is indistinctive.

The minimal expression of each of the clinical characteristics in the table has *not* been adequately defined so that various investigators cannot systematically and consistently reproduce each others' minimal findings. This results in major diagnostic problems in the identification of patients who have the minimal expression of the cutaneous phenotypes. Thus clinicians have great difficulty in clearly correlating cutaneous phenotypes to the genotypic status of each member of a FAMMM kindred. Further, clinicians do not have a high degree of accuracy in judging what nevus is an atypical nevus even when the nevi are larger than 4 or 5 mm in diameter. Grob et al.[11] have found relatively low sensitivity of the clinical examination (29%) for prediction of histologic dysplasia; that is, nevi with markers of histologic dysplasia are not necessarily atypical clinically. These investigators felt that the diagnosis of dysplastic nevi on the basis of clinical criteria alone is difficult and not reliable. Thus clinically, the demarcation line for small atypical nevi and normal nevi are not clear. In agreement with reduced expressivity of phenotype, some members of a FAMMM kindred may not express the phenotypes of many moles or atypical nevi and yet they can develop CMM *de novo*. In addition, they can have *none* of the three cutaneous phenotypes and yet develop the phenotype(s) of systemic nonmelanotic cancers of other anatomic sites as the only expression of their FAMMM genotype.[5,12,13] These phenomena should not be surprising because they represent some of the cardinal principles of medical genetics, namely, variable expressivity of phenotype and reduced gene penetrance.

V. HISTOLOGY OF ATYPICAL NEVI

The histology of the atypical nevus taken from FAMMM patients who have classic lesions shows cellular melanocytic atypia, architectural atypia, dermal fibrosis, angioneogenesis, and chronic lymphocytic inflammatory infiltrate. The histologic description of these criteria are enumerated in detail in another chapter of this book by Ruiter et al.[14] These findings were established by many investigators by simply sampling classic atypical nevi from florid examples of FAMMM kindreds who had many atypical nevi and probably, in some instances, CMM in their past history. As these histologic criteria are pushed to their minimum definition, their specificity becomes diminished. During the last decade, the histologic diagnosis of dysplastic nevus has become the linchpin in confirming the diagnosis of the FAMMM syndrome (hereditary dysplastic nevus syndrome). The same criteria are used in the diagnosis of the sporadic nevus syndrome; thus, the histology became the essential element in the clinical diagnosis. This evolution probably prompted the introduction of the new name for patients with this disorder, the atypical mole syndrome.[15] This histologic pivot is no longer secure as it suffers from the same inadequacies of defining the minimal expression of the clinical findings; that is, the definitions of the criteria breakdown in their specificity as they are placed closer to their minimal limits of expression.

The precise definition of histologic dysplasia for the confirmation of the clinical diagnosis of atypical nevi is still evolving, and its lower limits remain controversial. There are mixed opinions regarding the histopathologic features which are sufficient and required for the diagnosis of dysplastic nevi.[16,17] In the beginning of the histologic definition of atypical nevi in the FAMMM syndrome, melanocytic cellular atypia was included in the diagnostic criteria.[18,19,20] At the National Institutes of Health Consensus Conference, the group opinion was that architectural atypia could suffice for the diagnosis when attempting to establish the lower histologic limit of a AN from a patient who belonged to a kindred with the classic form of the FAMMM syndrome.[21] Murphy and Halpern[22] believe that the diagnosis of dysplastic nevi must include melanocytic cytologic atypia along with the other histologic criteria. Steijlen et al.,[23] in a statistical histologic study of AN from patients from a FAMMM group vs. AN from a "normal" control population, defined four histologic features: (1) junctional activity; (2) irregularity of melanocytic nests; (3) presence of dusty melanin pigment; and (4) size of melanocytic nuclei, which are associated statistically with dysplastic melanocytic nevi in individuals at a higher risk for the development of CMM. If more than one of these criteria are used, the accuracy of the histologic diagnosis becomes more discriminatory in separating AN in the FAMMM group from AN in the control group. A recent study using the same criteria has not verified these findings and found that the correlation between histologic atypia and risk of melanoma is too limited to be of general clinical use.[24] Each of these studies by reliable qualified investigative groups can only lead us to the conclusion that the definition of pathologic findings is still not secure. As always, defining the lower limits of histologic expression is exceedingly difficult. Perhaps extant histologic variation will prohibit morphology as an all encompassing discriminant. This insecurity is not limited to histology but is even more grossly apparent when defining the lower limits of what is acceptable clinical morphology of AN in adults. It becomes almost impossible in children where little data are present; therefore, no one has even addressed the issue of defining the clinical and histologic diagnosis of AN in children, especially prior to puberty.

VI. EVOLVING CONCEPTS

Within the past few years heretical concepts have slowly emerged. Ackerman[25] has recently proposed that the dysplastic nevus is a common nevus found in the normal population and is not diagnostic histologically of the dysplastic nevus syndrome. He believes that the dysplastic nevus should be called the common mole. The investigative group at the University of Utah has shown that if architectural atypia is used as the major criterion for diagnosis of dysplastic nevi, then 53% of normal spouse controls have one or more dysplastic nevi. Using the criterion of mild to moderate random nuclear atypia detected in 88% of their type 4 melanocytic lesions, the prevalence of dysplastic nevi is reduced to 47% of spouse controls. If a minimum clinical size limit of 5 mm is arbitrarily imposed as a diagnostic criterion, this will accommodate one fourth of all type 4A clinical lesions and will occur with a prevalence of 12% of the normal population. This latter figure is very close to the estimate often quoted for the prevalence of verified dysplastic nevi in the population. It should be remembered that the latter figure is based on the biased sampling of clinically atypical nevi seen in physicians' practices or large clinics where only the clinically abnormal or atypical lesions are excised for histologic examination.

Piepkorn[26] has proposed that the lentiginous pattern of intraepidermal melanocytic hyperplasia, with mild to moderate, random cytologic atypia, forms the conventional basis for the histologic definition of a dysplastic nevus and is actually the histologic pattern of a nevus in an active phase of radial growth. He believes that the lesser degrees of atypia, both architectural and cytologic, considered by many to be required for the diagnosis of dysplastic nevi, overlap with the histologic findings commonly seen in banal nevi and lentigines. In the initial discovery of the FAMMM syndrome it was thought that the diagnosis of this clinical disorder was made with the clinical recognition of the atypical nevi which was then confirmed by histologic examination. It then evolved that most dermatopathologists felt that "most dysplastic nevi can be diagnosed with certainty on histologic grounds alone."[27] We have now come full circle within a decade with the same investigators who now state that the clinical criteria alone may be all that is necessary for the adequate diagnosis of dysplastic nevus syndrome.[28] This of course is dependent upon what is meant by the "dysplastic nevus syndrome''. Are we speaking of the FAMMM syndrome (hereditary dysplastic nevus syndrome-HDNS) or are we speaking of the single patient who we have just seen who has not been investigated, the so-called sporadic DNS? This difference is important, as it dictates very divergent patterns of behavior for the physician who is confronted with his patient who has lots of moles with many of them large in size and ''funny-looking'', so-called atypical nevi.

VII. SPORADIC ATYPICAL MULTIPLE MOLE (SAMM) VS. THE FAMMM SYNDROME

The study of clinically atypical nevi has not been restricted to patients with only the FAMMM syndrome. The clinical and histologic investigations have also included patients with many atypical nevi who haven't had any in-depth investigations of relatives. The atypical nevi from the two groups have the same histologic characteristics. When confronted with such a patient we have to make decisions on diagnosis, treatment, and surveillance. Thus, all these patients received the designation of sporadic until proven otherwise. This brings into focus the definition of the hereditary and sporadic forms of the disorder. A review of the sporadic occurrence of atypical nevi in the population in most reported clinical studies shows that the investigators relied on the unverified family histories of their proband patients with atypical nevi and/or CMM. As has been shown, this procedure is associated with erroneous data at least two thirds of the time when it is obtained from a patient.[10] Probands in various studies of sporadic DNS have been used as the only historical resource in recalling the medical histories of their immediate family (first or possibly second degree relatives) for the occurrence of atypical nevi or malignant melanoma.[29-34] These studies have not determined if the sporadic patients have a genetic trait as they have not had any in-depth genealogical evaluations. It should be remembered that sporadic is an operational term and is not the opposite of hereditary and, therefore, is not *non*hereditary. The definition of the designation FAMMM and sporadic is important to the clinician as it emphasizes major differences in the medial investigation of these patients, the therapeutic procedures, and the program of cancer surveillance.

The FAMMM designation of a patient mandates genetic counseling of the proband and his kindred. This autosomal dominant inherited trait indicates possible high risk for CMM especially if any members of the kindred have had CMM. In addition, there may be a high risk for primary systemic cancer of other anatomic sites which can only be established by an investigation of the occurrence pattern of systemic cancer(s) in the extended pedigree of the kindred (especially beyond the second degree relatives of the proband). This aspect of the FAMMM syndrome has been verified by Bergman et al.[12] in nine Dutch kindreds and shows the heterogeneity of the primary nonmelanoma systemic cancer expression in that only three of the nine kindreds showed a pancreatic cancer occurrence that was 28 times the national Dutch incidence data. The genetic nature of FAMMM pattern of systemic cancer is even more apparent with the absence of colon cancer in the same three pedigrees. For every pancreatic cancer in the Netherlands, colon cancer is five times more prevalent. Lynch and Fusaro[35] have recently updated the original FAMMM kindred reported by Lynch and Krush[8] in which three members of a small FAMMM kindred have died from adenocarcinoma of the pancreas. All three cancer victims, who were gene carriers of the FAMMM trait, were within a first degree relationship and lived in different geographical areas. This would of course suggest that the genetic pattern in this FAMMM kindred was similar to the genotype reported by Bergman et al.[12] in the Netherlands. Other FAMMM kindreds reported by us[5] have an increased occurrence of different patterns of systemic cancer of other anatomic sites in addition to the increased risk for CMM.

This heterogeneity of the FAMMM syndrome with respect to systemic cancer is also

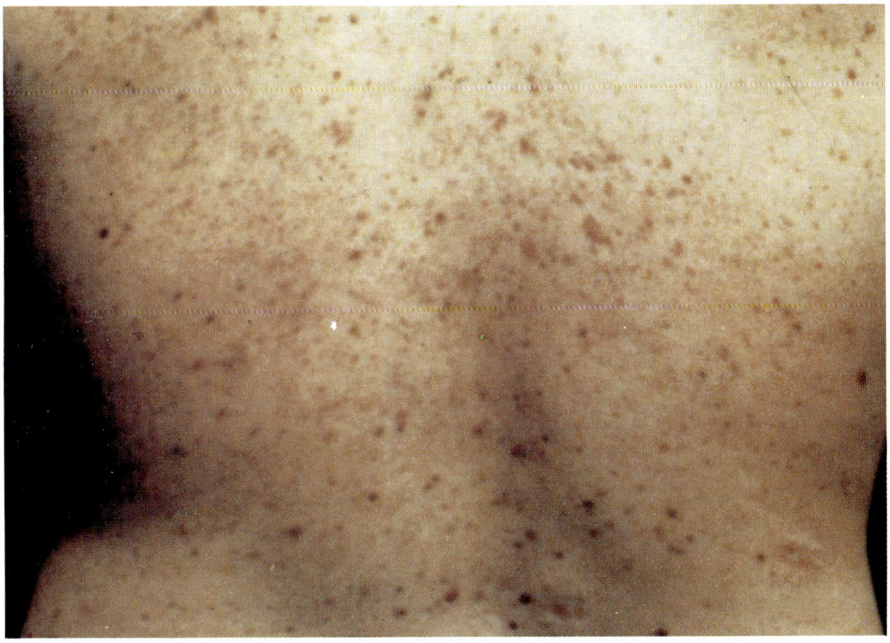

PLATE 1A.

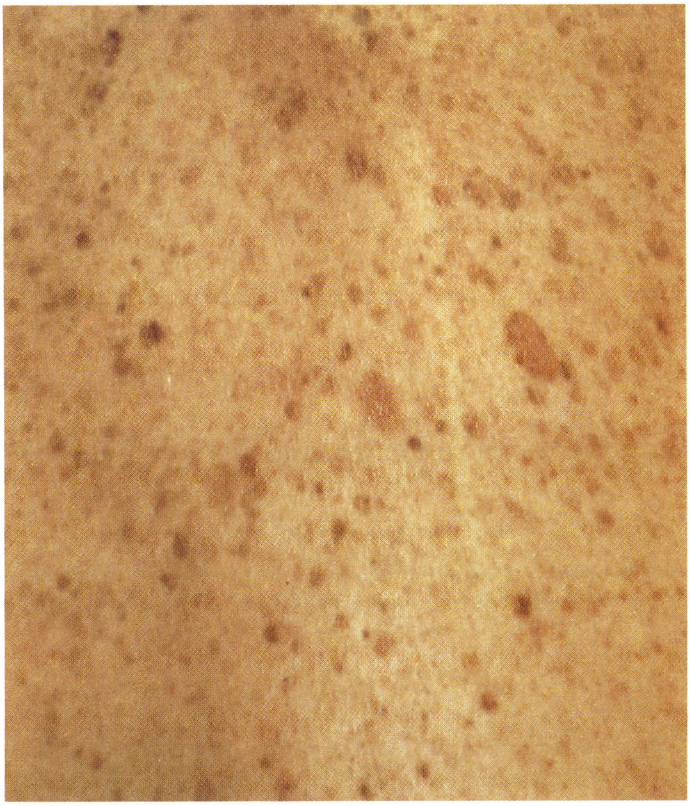

PLATE 1B.

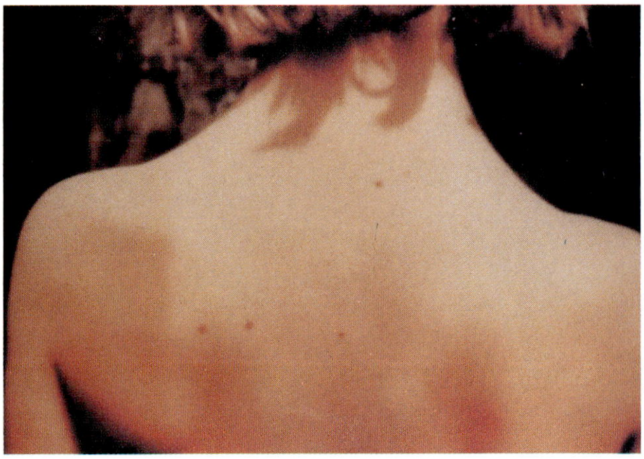

PLATE 2A.

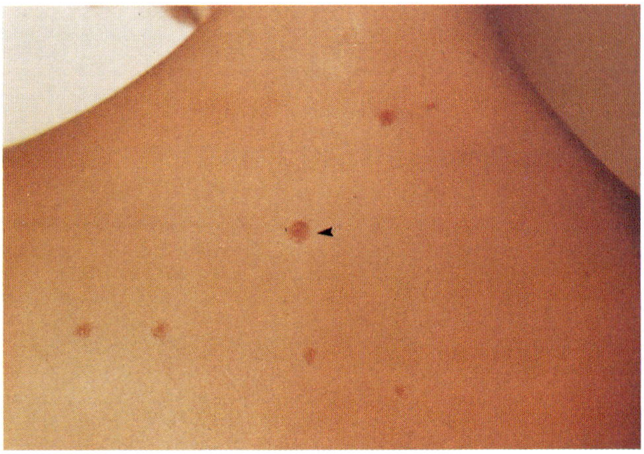

PLATE 2B.

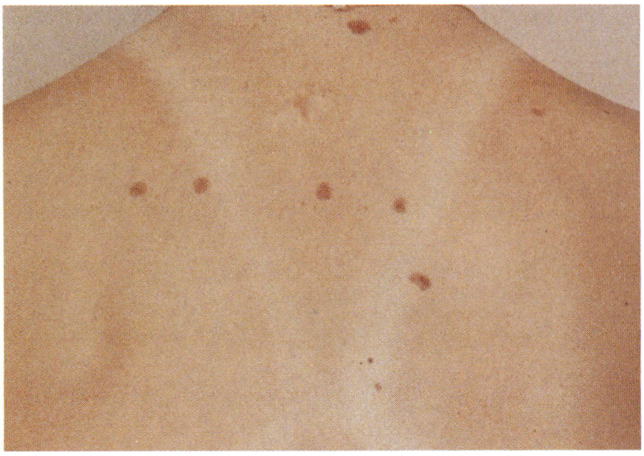

PLATE 2C.

manifested in the genetic expression of the cutaneous phenotypes seen in such kindreds; that is, the expression of the cutaneous phenotypes is markedly different in the various FAMMM kindreds with some kindreds showing no evidence of CMM, but they do have the usual florid expression of atypical moles and large number of total body moles. Therefore, the heterogeneity seen in the systemic cancer expression is not confined to that phenotypic expression of systemic cancer(s) but is universal and also expressed in the cutaneous phenotypes of atypical moles, the total number of body moles, and the expression of CMM in the kindreds. Thus, the diagnosis of the FAMMM syndrome puts into operation a genealogical investigation of the kindred which is only limited by the knowledge of the names of distant members of the kindred. The genealogical investigation should be extended into the distant relatives of the kindred as far as possible to inform all who carry the high risk for cancer. The FAMMM diagnosis also sets up a cancer surveillance program which is not only concerned with CMM but moreover is specific for the particular systemic cancer(s) pattern of each kindred under investigation. The frequency and diagnostic direction of these specific investigations will be dependent upon the findings in the extended pedigree in order to be cost effective. This means that if a genetically integral primary systemic cancer(s) is found in any particular kindred, then a surveillance program can be initiated and targeted for that particular organ system which has been implicated. Given the high risk status, one is in a better position to increase cancer diagnostic yield and thereby approach cost effectiveness.

The designation of a patient with multiple atypical moles and high total mole counts as a sporadic atypical multiple mole (SAMM) patient initiates a very different course of events in the investigative, therapeutic, and surveillance care of the individual with a SAMM designation. This latter designation implies the following numerous definitions of the operational term sporadic: (1) inadequate family history and examination of the patient and his kindred; (2) until more information is obtained, the observed clinical manifestations of a SAMM patient may be due to incomplete penetrance, variable expressivity, and a spectrum of heterogeneity of the FAMMM genotype; (3) there may be a lack of adequate genetic information due to small size of the proband's kindred; (4) the occurrence of the dubious father phenomenon; (5) a different genotype; (6) a fresh germinal mutation of the FAMMM genotype; and (7) a true phenocopy of the FAMMM syndrome. All of these alternatives necessitate genealogical and medical investigations of our SAMM patients and their relatives. In addition, in the last two alternatives, a follow-up of the proband's progeny for at least two generations is necessary to establish with some security the identification of either a fresh germinal mutation of the FAMMM genotype with its possible cancer risks for the progeny or a true phenocopy without any additive risk for the progeny. Thus the investigation of the SAMM patient requires a surveillance for malignant melanoma dependent upon personal risk factors, but more importantly, a concerted effort by the patient's physician to investigate the kindred to elicit further genealogical data to either establish or reject the concept of inheritance with not only increased risk for CMM but also possible risk for primary systemic cancers of other organ systems.

VIII. CONCLUSIONS

The concept of hereditary malignant melanoma in the form of the FAMMM syndrome is still evolving from a very simplistic concept to what now appears to be a very complex disorder(s), which still has many unknown facets to be uncovered. The genetic trait of the FAMMM syndrome has been present for eons, but its failure to be recognized by dermatologists and oncologists is probably due to our historical lack of acceptance of the extent of hereditary cancer. In general, this in turn is due to our mind set from our cultural philosophy, of the myth that all men are created equal. It is apparent from reviewing investigations reported in the literature that there are extremely few acceptable in-depth genealogical studies. Because of these inadequacies, many premature conclusions have been made concerning the FAMMM syndrome. Even more inappropriate data have been assembled concerning SAMM patients. It is clear from the investigative work of the past decade that we are having difficulty defining the limits of the spectrum of the disorder both cutaneously and histologically. The qualitative and quantitative limits of the expression of systemic cancer are even more unknown. If genealogical research is done properly on this disorder, we can except from present and future research efforts further changes in our concepts of the FAMMM's etiological and pathogenetic mechanisms which will ultimately lead us to better care of our SAMM and FAMMM patients.

REFERENCES

1. **Lynch, H. T., Frichot, B. C., and Lynch, J. F.,** Familial atypical multiple mole melanoma syndrome, *J. Med. Genet.*, 15, 352, 1978.
2. **Clark, W. H., Jr., Reimer, R. R., Greene, M. H., Ainsworth, A. M., and Mastrangelo, M. J.,** Origin of familial malignant melanomas from heritable melanocytic lesions: 'the B-K mole syndrome', *Arch. Dermatol.*, 114, 732, 1978.
3. **Bergman, W., Palan, A., and Went, L. N.,** Clinical and genetic studies in six Dutch kindreds with the dysplastic nevus syndrome, *Ann. Hum. Genet.*, 50, 249, 1986.
4. **Meyer, L. J., Piepkorn, M. W., Sechter, S. A., Cannon-Albright, L. A., Bishop, D. T., Zone, J. J., and Skolnick, M. H.,** Genetic and epidemiologic evaluation of dysplastic nevi, *Pigm. Cell. Res.*, Suppl. 1, 144, 1988.
5. **Lynch, H. T., Fusaro, R. M., Kimberling, W. J., and Lynch, J. F.,** Familial atypical multiple mole melanoma (FAMMM) syndrome: segregation analysis, *J. Med. Genet.*, 20, 342, 1983.
6. **Norris, W.,** A case of fungoid disease, *Edin. Med. Surg. J.*, 16, 562, 1820.
7. **Cawley, E. P.,** Genetic aspects of malignant melanoma, *Arch. Dermatol. Syphilol.*, 65, 440, 1952.
8. **Lynch, H. T. and Krush, A. J.,** Heredity and malignant melanoma: implications for cancer detection, *Can. Med. Assoc. J.*, 99, 17, 1968.
9. **Lynch, H. T. and Fusaro, R. M.,** *Cancer Associated Genodermatoses*, Van Nostrand Reinhold, New York, 1982.
10. **Lynch, H. T., Follett, K. L., Lynch, P. M., Albano, W. A., Mailliard, J. A., and Pierson, R. L.,** Family history in an oncology clinic: implications for cancer genetics, *JAMA*, 242, 1268, 1979.
11. **Grob, J. J., Andrac, L., Romano, M. H., et al.,** Dysplastic naevus in nonfamilial melanoma: a clinicopathological study of 101 cases, *Br. J. Dermatol.*, 118, 745, 1988.
12. **Bergman, W., Watson, P., deJong, J., Lynch, H. T., and Fusaro, R. M.,** Systemic cancer and the FAMMM syndrome, *Br. J. Cancer*, 61, 932, 1990.
13. **Lynch, H. T. and Fusaro, R. M.,** Pancreatic cancer and the familial atypical multiple mole melanoma (FAMMM) syndrome, *Pancreas*, 1990, submitted.
14. **Ruiter, D. J., Steylen, P. M., van der Wiel-Miexenbeek, J., Henzen-Logmans, S. C., Mooi, W. J., Bergman, W., and Scheffer, E.,** Histopathological criteria required for the diagnosis of familial dysplastic nevi, in *Hereditary Malignant Melanoma*, Lynch, H. T. and Fusaro, R. M., Eds., CRC Press, Boca Raton, FL, 1991, chap. 2.
15. **Kopf, A. W., Friedman, R. J., and Riegel, D. S.,** Atypical mole syndrome, *J. Am. Acad. Dermatol.*, 22, 118, 1990.
16. **Seywright, M. M., Doherty, V. R., and MacKie, R. M.,** Proposed alternative terminology and subclassification of so-called dysplastic nevi, *J. Clin. Pathol.*, 39, 189, 1986.
17. **Ackerman, A. B. and Mihara, I.,** Dysplasia, dysplastic melanocytes, dysplastic nevi, the dysplastic nevus syndrome, and the relation between dysplastic nevi and malignant melanomas, *Hum. Pathol.*, 16, 87, 1985.
18. **Elder, D. E., Goldman, L. I., Goldman, S. C., et al.,** Dysplastic nevus syndrome, a phenotypic association of sporadic cutaneous melanoma, *Cancer*, 46, 1787, 1980.
19. **English, D. R., Menz, J., Heenan, P. J., et al.,** The dysplastic nevus syndrome in patients with cutaneous malignant melanoma in Western Australia, *Med. J. Aust.*, 145, 194, 1986.
20. **Clark, W. H., Jr., Elder, D. E., Guerry, D., et al.,** A study of tumor progression, the precursor lesion of superficial spreading and nodular melanoma, *Hum. Pathol.*, 15, 1147, 1984.
21. National Institute of Health Consensus Conference, Precursors to malignant melanoma, *JAMA*, 251, 1864, 1984.

22. **Murphy, G. F. and Halpern, G. F.,** Dysplastic melanocytic nevi: normal variants or melanoma precursors?, *Arch. Dermatol.,* 126, 519, 1990.
23. **Steijlen, P. M., Bergman, W., Hermans, J., Scheffer, E., van Vlkoten, W. A., and Ruiter, D. J.,** The efficacy of histopathological criteria required for diagnosing dysplastic naevi, *Histopathology,* 12, 289, 1988.
24. **Ahmed, I., Piepkorn, M. W., Rabkin, M. S., Meyer, L. J., Feldkamp, M., Goldgar, D. E., Skolnick, M. H., and Zone, J. J.,** Histopathologic characteristics of dysplastic nevi: limited association of conventional histologic criteria with melanoma risk group, *J. Am. Acad. Dermatol.,* 22, 727, 1990.
25. **Ackerman, A. B.,** What naevus is dysplastic, a syndrome, and the commonest precursor of malignant melanoma? A riddle and an answer, *Histopathology,* 13, 241, 1988.
26. **Piepkorn, M.,** A hypothesis incorporating the histologic characteristics of dysplastic nevi into the normal biological development of melanocytic nevi, *Arch. Dermatol.,* 126, 514, 1990.
27. **Elder, D. E., Greene, M. H., Guerry, D. IV, Kraemer, K. H., and Clark, W. H., Jr.,** The dysplastic nevus syndrome: our definition, *Am. J. Dermatopathol.,* 4, 455, 1982.
28. **Cooke, K. R., Spears, G. F. S., Elder, D. E., and Greene, M. H.,** Dysplastic naevi in a population based study, *Cancer,* 63, 1240, 1989.
29. **Nordlund, J. J., Kirkwook, J., Forget, B. M., et al.,** Demographic study of clinically atypical nevi in patients with melanoma and comparison subjects, *Cancer Res.,* 45, 1855, 1985.
30. **Holly, E. A., Kelly, F. W., Shpall, S. N., and Chiu, S. H.,** Number of melanocytic nevi as a major risk factor for malignant melanoma, *J. Am. Acad. Dermatol.,* 17, 459, 1987.
31. **MacKie, R. M., Freudenberger, T., and Aitchison, T. C.,** Personal risk factor chart for cutaneous melanoma, *Lancet,* 2, 487, 1989.
32. **Kraemer, K. H. and Greene, M. H.,** Dysplastic nevus syndrome. Familial and sporadic precursors of cutaneous melanoma, *Dermatol. Clin.,* 3, 225, 1985.
33. **Kraemer, K. H., Tucker, M., Tarone, R., Elder, D. E., and Clark, W. H., Jr.,** Risk of cutaneous melanoma in dysplastic nevus syndrome types A and B, *N. Engl. J. Med.,* 315, 1615, 1986.
34. **Rahbari, H. and Mehregan, A. H.,** Sporadic atypical mole syndrome, *Arch. Dermatol.,* 117, 329, 1981.
35. **Lynch, H. T. and Fusaro, R. M.,** Pancreatic cancer and the familial atypical multiple mole melanoma (FAMMM) syndrome, *Pancreas,* 6, in press.

Chapter 3

THE FAMMM SYNDROME IN THE NETHERLANDS

W. Bergman, A. van Haeringen, and L. N. Went

TABLE OF CONTENTS

I. INTRODUCTION

A. ASCERTAINMENT OF FAMILIES

In February 1982 the Pigmented Lesions Clinic (PLC) of the Department of Dermatology of Leiden University Hospital was established, facilitating studies on familial melanoma. The kindreds were detected through intensive case finding among melanoma patients attending the surgical oncology department of the hospital. Both new melanoma patients and melanoma patients during follow-up were interrogated on two successive occasions about the presence of melanomas in relatives. If there was a positive response, the patient was given a questionnaire; on the basis of these data in the first instance all first and second degree relatives were requested to attend the PLC for careful analysis of their skin. All family members were interviewed and examined by the same dermatologist. At the first visit an extended questionnaire was filled out concerning sun exposure, skin type, use of drugs, exposure to environmental agents, and concomitant diseases. The number of nevi were counted and the clinical characteristics and localization described. All individuals were photographed and suspicious lesions were removed. Details on the histopathological criteria that were used to diagnose dysplastic nevi can be found in Chapter 5.

In the first few months after the establishment of the PLC we found evidence of familial melanoma in about 18 melanoma patients, some of which appeared to have multiple family members affected with melanoma, while others had only one other family member affected with melanoma. At this point we did not have information yet on the presence of atypical nevi in melanoma patients or their family members. The 18 melanoma patients were from a group of 186 patients who were registered for follow-up; their (stage 1) melanomas were diagnosed between 1973 and 1982 (10.7%).

Not being able to investigate these families all at once, we started to ascertain those families in which more than two melanomas were reported to occur. Thus we found ten families, six of which have been reported earlier elsewhere.[1] The ascertainment of these families is biased in that they were the easiest accessible. In all ten families several family members showing atypical nevi were found validating the diagnosis of the FAMMM syndrome. In this chapter these families will be discussed and analyzed.

Later we studied seven more independent families, showing only two family members affected with melanoma at that time; these families have not yet been analyzed completely, although they have been investigated clinically. There do not seem to be obvious clinical differences among the 17 families, but the more recent families tend to be smaller, which might be an explanation for the finding of "only" two melanoma patients.

B. CLUSTERING OF FAMILIES

All families were from the region of Leiden and lived within a distance of 50 km from the hospital. Figure 1 shows the clustering of FAMMM families: five of the ten families were from the same coastal fishing village, and three came from a village 20 km from Leiden in a rural region. As far back as 1830 we did not find common ancestors among these eight families. One family came from The Hague and one originated from Utrecht. The "cluster villages" seemed to have in common families that were affected, who had lived there for many generations. In addition, these villages had an orthodox religious population with large families and strong family ties. Individuals in these families rarely moved to other places. These circumstances facilitated genetic studies. It is not clear if this clustering of the FAMMM trait can be totally explained by the so-called "founder effect", which means that many different families in a certain restricted area have had a common ancestor.

In conclusion, eight FAMMM families were clustered in two villages close to Leiden, which according to us is probably explained by the founder effect. It should not be excluded that elsewhere in the Netherlands other unrelated families with the FAMMM syndrome occurred.

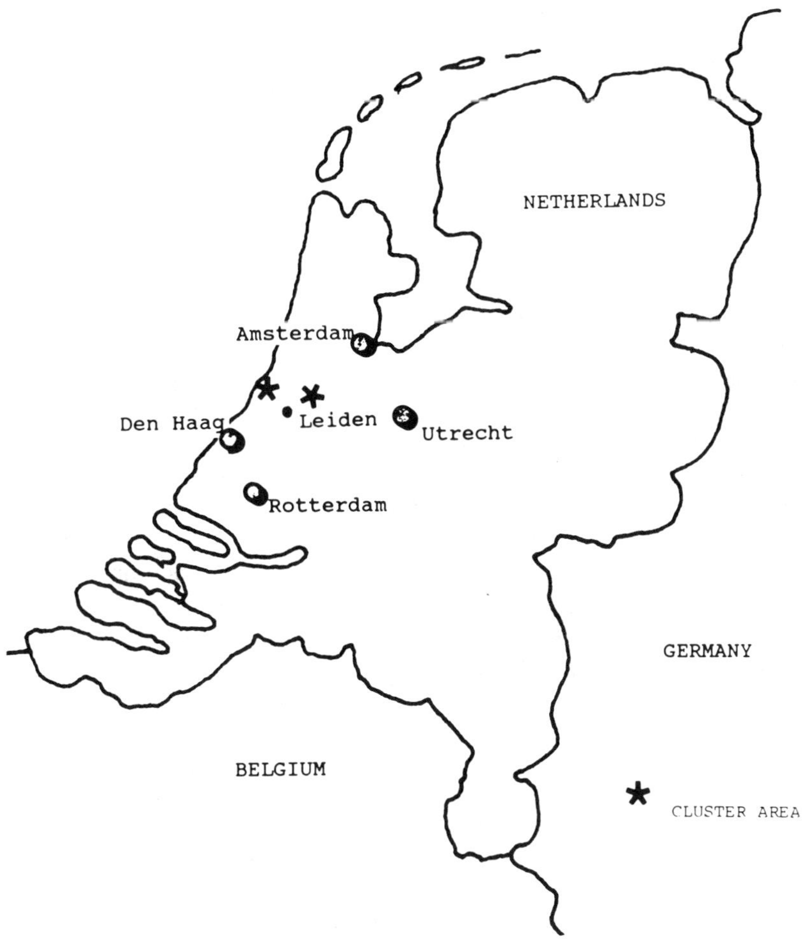

FIGURE 1. Clustering of FAMMM families in the Netherlands.

C. MODE OF INHERITANCE

Most investigators studying pedigrees with the FAMMM syndrome came to the conclusion that the condition was autosomal dominantly inherited with usually 40 to 50% of the children of affected individuals being proven gene carriers themselves.[2-4] However, arguments against autosomal dominant inheritance were presented by Happle and co-workers who suggested polygenic inheritance.[5-7] Recently, a report was published in which it was claimed that the gene responsible for the FAMMM syndrome was located at the top of chromosome 1*p* in six American FAMMM families.[8] This claim could not be confirmed in a study from the Netherlands, which will be discussed later (see Section II.D). Genetic heterogeneity could be a possible explanation for these divergent results. It should be remembered, however, that linkage studies for the localization of a gene can be incorrectly interpreted, when this gene is nonpenetrant in a considerable number of individuals, as is the case with the FAMMM syndrome. Proof of this nonpenetrance will be presented in Section II.B.

II. THE DUTCH FAMMM FAMILIES

A. THE FAMILY MEMBERS

In Figures 2 to 11 the pedigrees of the ten melanoma-prone kindreds that were studied in detail are reproduced. In all families individuals with dysplastic nevi were found. The

LEGEND FOR FIGURES 2 TO 11

Pedigrees of the 10 Dutch families with FAMMM syndrome.

investigated — deceased

clinical FAMMM moles — FAMMM moles (path. verified)

melanoma — proband with melanoma and FAMMM moles

total number of family members (affected or at risk) in the ten pedigrees as presented in these figures was 540. In pedigree 1 the unaffected daughter of II-9, who married into the family, was herself a member of a not yet fully studied melanoma family. Pedigree 2 will be discussed in detail later (see Section II.E). In pedigree 5 the spouse of II-5 showed several clinically dysplastic nevi, so that possibly both husband and wife are gene carriers. The children of this couple have been left out of the genetic analysis.

Of all 534 persons older than 10 years, in total 428 were seen at our outpatient department. Forty-six individuals (10%) did not attend and 60 individuals were dead at the time of the investigation (causes of death: malignant melanoma of the skin, 16; cancer at various sites, 29; other causes, 15). Of the 29 individuals who died of malignancies other than melanoma, 23 were found in three of the ten pedigrees. Details on the different types of cancer found in these families can be found in Chapter 1.

Apart from the patients with melanoma, in our ten families 65 individuals had multiple atypical nevi which were histologically investigated, thus verifying the clinical diagnosis. Another 58 people showed several apparently dysplastic nevi, with such a quiet appearance that excision to date was not thought to be necessary. These patients are indicated in the pedigree as cases of clinical dysplastic nevi.

In Table 1 a numerical breakdown is given of the investigated (living) individuals, divided into patients with melanoma, with dysplastic nevi, obligate gene carriers, and individuals with no abnormalities. We considered "obligate" gene carriers only individuals who themselves did not have any suspicious nevi, but who had one or more children with melanoma or histologically verified dysplastic nevi or at least two children with clinically dysplastic nevi.

B. GENETIC STUDIES OF THE TEN FAMILIES

The data from the ten families and a study of their pedigrees seem to indicate clearly that a dominant gene with variable expressivity and incomplete penetrance is responsible both for the occurrence of malignant melanoma of the skin and for the presence of dysplastic nevi. Vertical transmission of the gene through three consecutive generations occurred in six pedigrees and through two consecutive generations in four pedigrees. More or less equal numbers of males and females were affected in the ten pedigrees and father to son transmission occurred 14 times in ten pedigrees.

From the data presented in Table 1 it can be seen that at least 187 of 428 investigated individuals from ten pedigrees must carry the gene (43.7%).

Since the initial requirement to undertake a family study was the minimal presence of three individuals with melanoma, we have to deduct from the number of melanoma patients three index cases per family (10 × 3 = 30) to correct for bias of ascertainment. Twelve of these 30 were dead at the time of our study, so that of the 37 living melanoma patients from Table 2, 18 have to be deducted. After this correction we find 169 gene carriers in a total group of 410 investigated persons. We found no abnormalities in 241 family members. On the basis of dominant inheritance, 321 of all investigated 410 individuals had an *a priori* risk of 50% to have inherited the gene, 82 a risk of 25%, and 7 a risk of only $12^1/_2$%. Thus

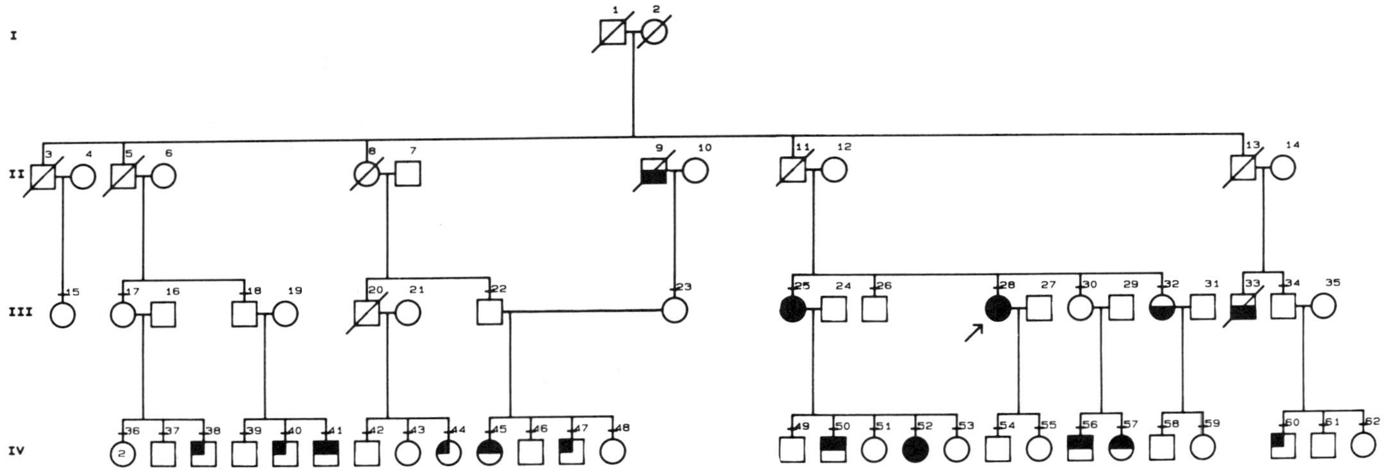

FIGURE 2. Family VBE-1.

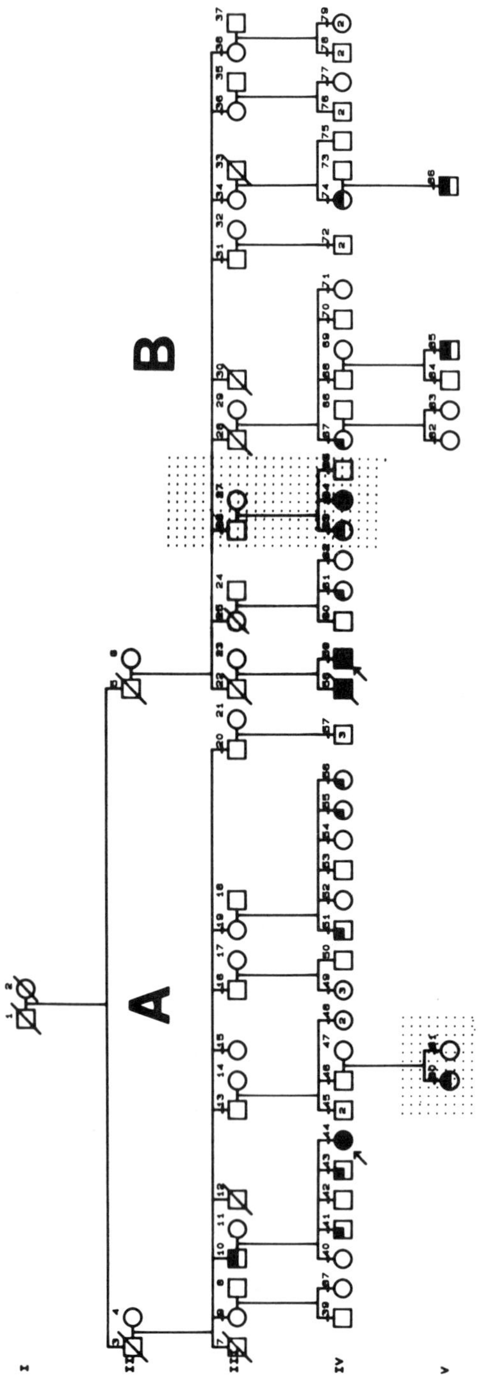

FIGURE 3. Family VDB-2.

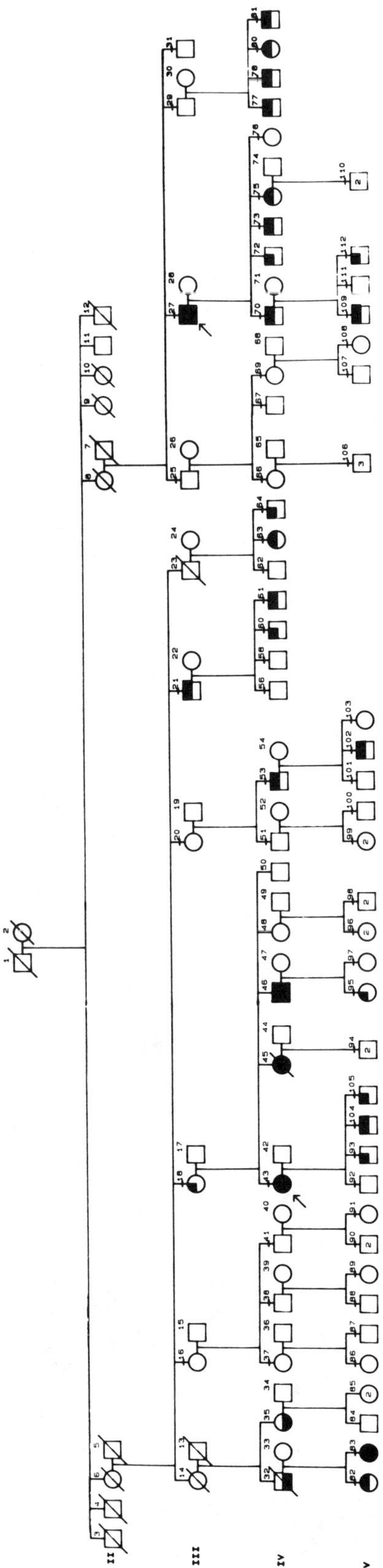

FIGURE 4. Family H-3.

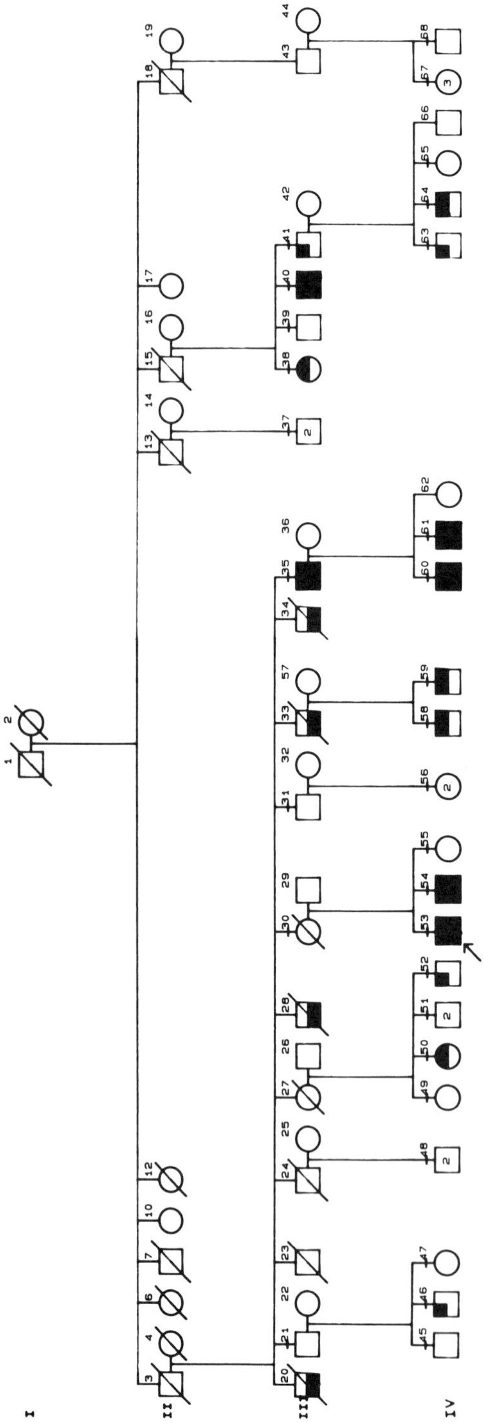

FIGURE 5. Family F-4.

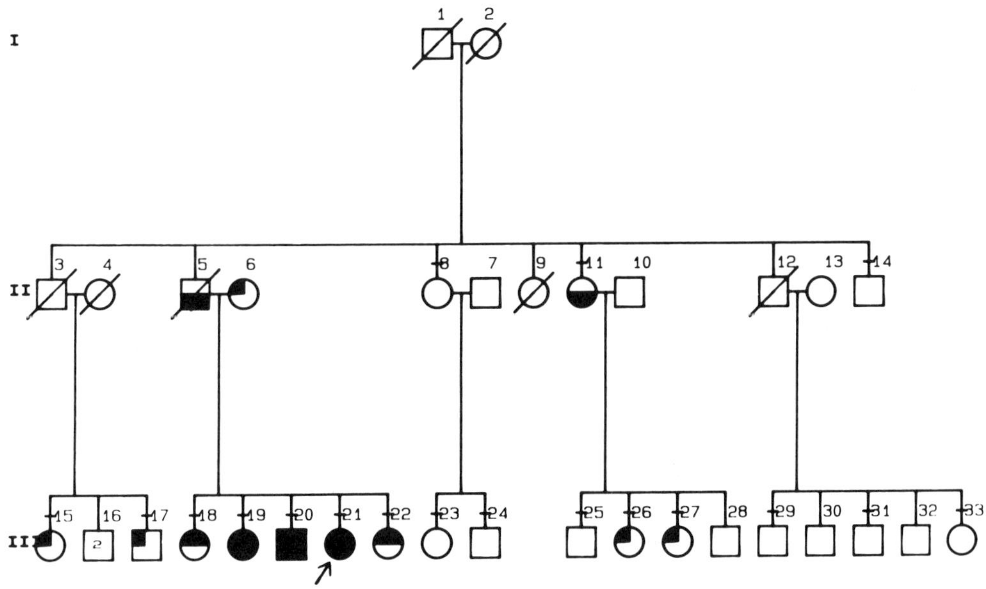

FIGURE 6. Family J-5.

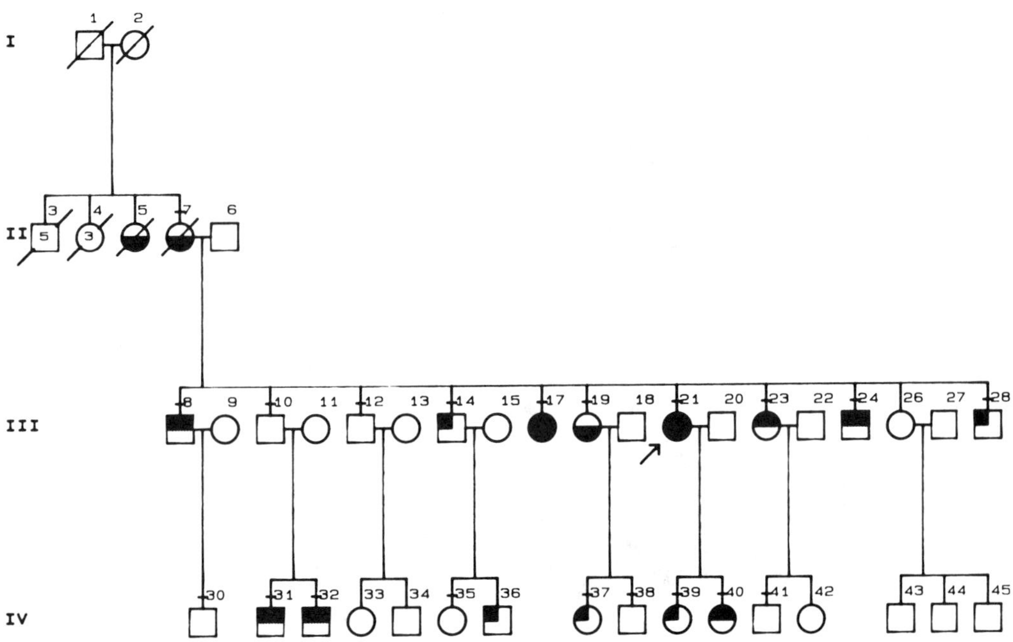

FIGURE 7. Family Z-6.

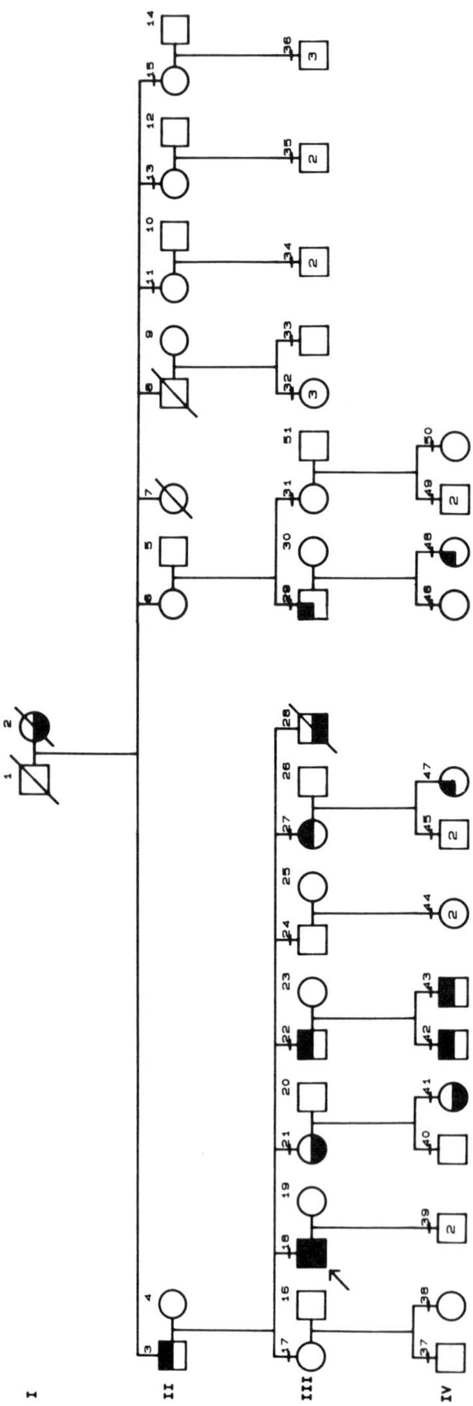

FIGURE 8. Family M-7.

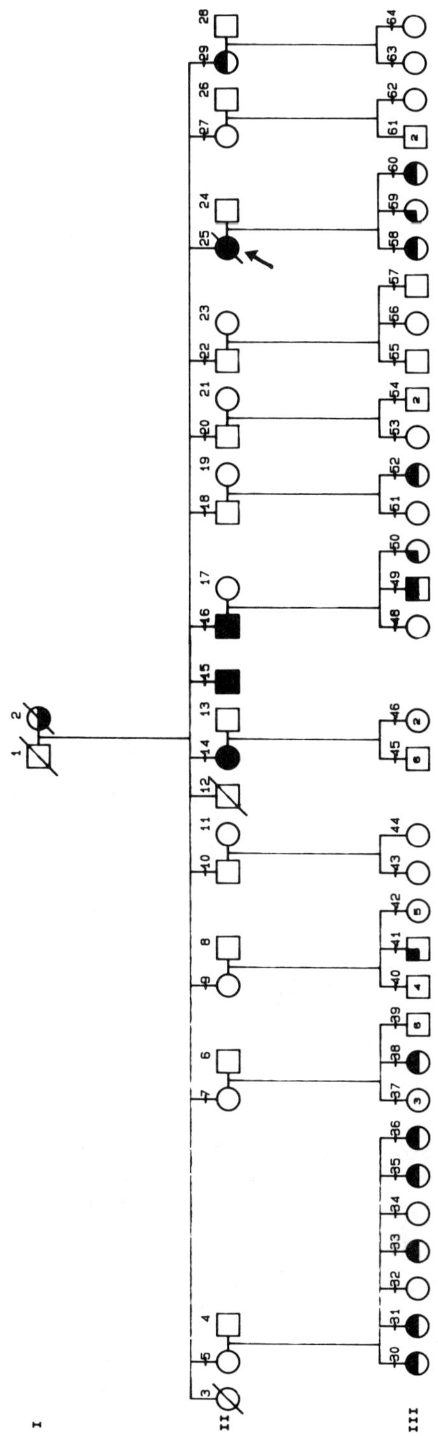

FIGURE 9. Family Z-10.

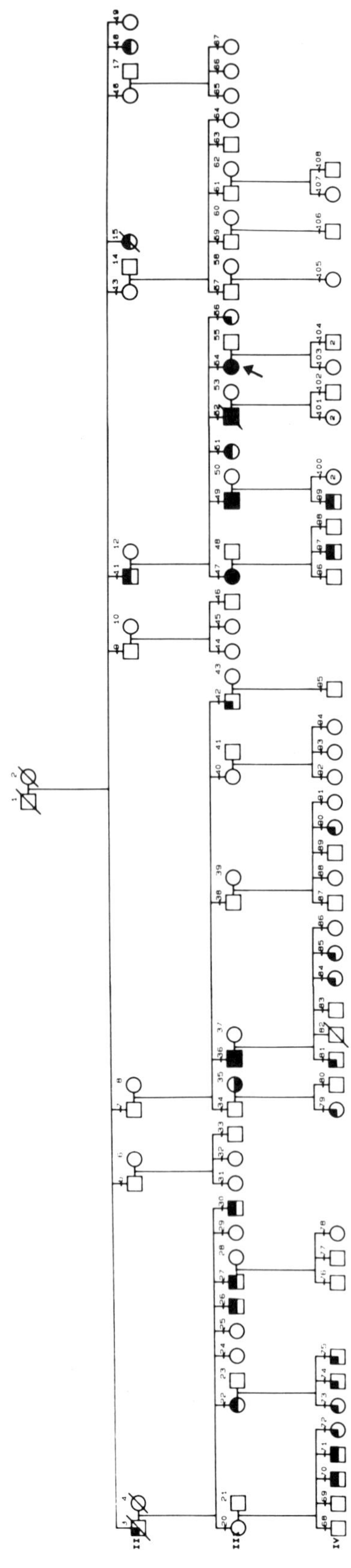

FIGURE 10. Family Ey-14.

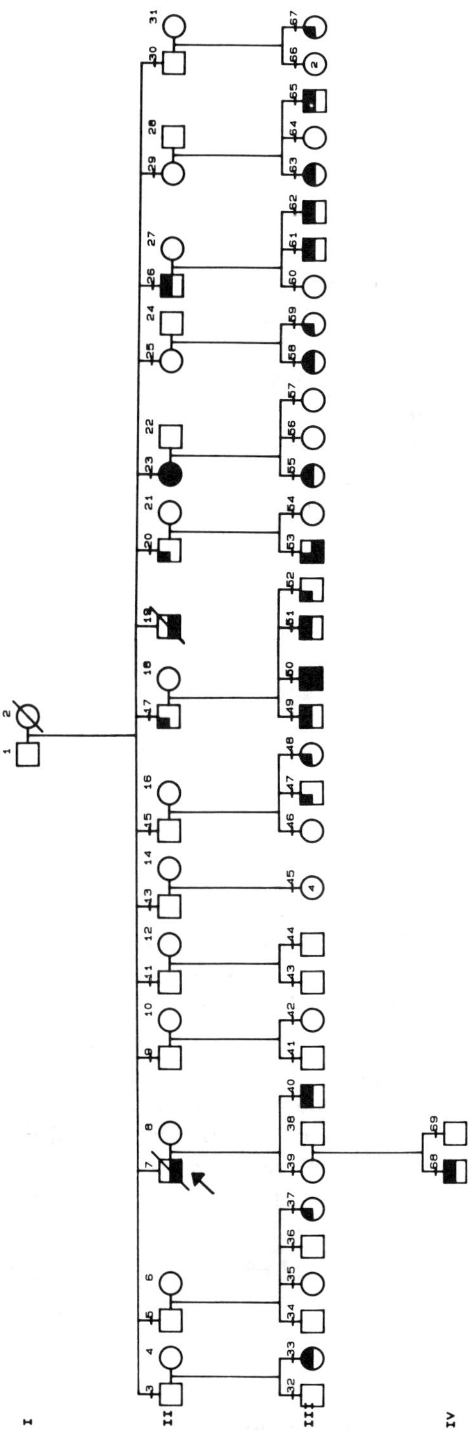

FIGURE 11. Family Ba-19.

TABLE 1
Occurrence of Affected and Unaffected Individuals in Ten Pedigrees

	Number of living investigated individuals with				
	Melanoma	FAMMM moles	Obligate gene carriers	No abnormality	Not investigated
Number	37 (19)[a]	123	27	241	46
Mean age (years)	38.4	22.8	54.3	26.8	
Range	16—68	11—74	32—74	11—70	

Note: 187 gene carriers (169); [a] 428 investigated individuals (410).[a]

[a] The figures in parenthesis are after correction for bias of ascertainment.

TABLE 2
Lod Scores for Linkage Between DNS and Marker Loci on the Short Arm of Chromosome 1

Locus	Regional localization	Recombinations fraction (0)					N	cM
		0.01	0.10	0.20	0.30	0.40		
DNF15S1	1*p*36.3	−5.06	−2.47	−1.07	−0.39	−0.08	23	12
D1Z2	1*p*36.3	−5.91	−3.51	−1.73	−0.76	−0.25	25	16
RH	1*p*34	−17.24	−6.98	−2.80	−0.96	−0.27	53	23
FUCA1	1*p*34	−6.05	−2.44	−0.97	−0.33	−0.07	34	12
D1S17	1*p*31-pter	−6.75	−3.63	−1.62	−0.62	−0.12	25	18
D1S57	1*p*	−6.27	−4.74	−3.12	−1.61	−0.60	29	27
PGM1	1*p*22.1	−3.82	−2.10	−0.25	+0.09	+0.14	18	11
PND	1*p* 36	−6.00	−2.38	−1.14	−0.50	−0.18	19	13

Note: N, number of informative meioses; cM, centiMorgans definitely excluded on either side of the tested marker, assuming lodscores of −2 or less as definite proof for exclusion; DNS gene frequency 0.003; life time penetrance 85%.

one should expect, again on the assumption of dominant inheritance, that about 182 ($^1/_2 \times$ 321) + ($^1/_4 \times$ 82) + ($^1/_8 \times$ 7) individuals should have inherited the abnormal gene for FAMMM, whereas 169 were recognized as such (92%). Among these 169 there were 27 who were phenotypically entirely normal, but who were obligate gene carriers on the basis of their position in the pedigree. This would give a minimal nonpenetrance rate of 0.16, but the actual figure will be higher since among the 241 persons with no abnormalities more gene carriers are likely to occur. It is obvious that nonpenetrance can only be proven in older generations; the children of gene carriers have to be old enough to show signs of the syndrome. This is confirmed by the mean age of the obligate gene carriers: 54.3 years, while the mean age of the unaffected persons was 26.8 years. It is to be expected that a number of persons may still develop dysplastic nevi or a melanoma at an older age.

In summary our pedigrees reveal an autosomal dominant mode of inheritance with a nonpenetrance rate of more than 0.16.

C. LINKAGE STUDIES

Linkage studies using polymorphic markers were carried out on six of our ten families.[9] We decided to focus on the short arm of chromosome 1 to confirm or reject the reported loose linkage with the rhesus locus (chromosome 1p34) reported by Greene et al.[3] and the strong positive lodscore data concerning chromosome 1p36 recently reported by Bale et al.[8]

The following erythrocyte serum markers were tested: rhesus blood group (RH), located at 1p34, α-1-fucosidase (FUCA1), located at 1p34, phosphoglucomutase-1 (PGM1), located at 1p34. Also tested were the following polymorphic DNA probes: pH_3H_2 (DNF15S1), located at 1p36.3; p1-79 (D1Z2), a hypervariable probe located at 1p36.3; pYNZ-2 (D1S57), a variable number of tandem repeats (VNTR) probe located between RG and PGM1; p3-18 (D1S17), located at 1p31.

Additionally, we have very recently added to the panel the probe pJA110 (PND) (located at 1p36) which particular probe revealed a very high lodscore in the American study by Bale et al.[8] Together, this panel of eight polymorphic markers completely spans the short arm of chromosome 1.

Linkage analysis was carried out using the LINKAGE programs. The FAMMM gene frequency was estimated at 0.003 with a lifetime penetrance of 85% as was found in our families and described in Section II.B. As can be seen in Table 2, RH yields a strong negative lod score for all recombination frequencies, allowing exclusion of 23 centiMorgans on either side of the marker. Moreover, all the other seven markers gave negative lod scores. The combined linkage data thus definitely exclude the FAMMM gene from the short arm of chromosome 1 in our families.

Following our negative results in the chromosome 1p region, we will continue our search for the "Dutch" version of the FAMMM gene. At present, after testing more than 50 polymorphic DNA probes throughout the genome, no significant/suggestive positive lod scores have been found, whereas about 70% of the genome could be excluded from harboring the gene.

D. DETAILS ON PATIENTS WHO DEVELOPED A MELANOMA

In the ten families, 42 persons (16 males, 26 females) with 55 melanomas could be reviewed. Data on nine of the ten families with respect to the impact of screening have been reported recently.[10] All cases were verified pathologically. Twenty-six of the 42 melanoma patients (60%) showed clinically the cutaneous phenotype of the FAMMM syndrome, and in 24 this diagnosis was histologically verified. Sixteen patients died of melanoma before the time of our study. The average age at death was 47.1 years (ages of death ranging between 18 and 66 years). One boy (not included in the study) died assumedly from melanoma at the age of 8 years (in 1930), but confirmation was not available. Eleven of the 42 persons developed more than one primary melanoma (26%). Twenty-one melanomas had been diagnosed before the start of the screening program (category A). The average age of the patients whose first melanoma was detected before the start of the screening was 47.1 years. To date 34 newly diagnosed melanomas have occurred in 26 family members. Twelve were detected at the initial examination of the families (category B, average age 41.1 years), and 24 melanomas were found during the course of follow-up studies (category C, average age 28.9 years).

The age at diagnosis and the developmental stage of melanomas in the three categories are shown in Table 3. Melanomas *in situ* were found in 1 out of 21 melanomas in category A, in 3 of the 12 in category B, and in 8 of the 24 in category C. The average thickness of the invasive melanomas in the three categories was 1.88, 0.81, and 0.51 mm, respectively. The average age at diagnosis of the melanomas in these categories (47.1, 41.1, 28.9) did not differ significantly ($p = 0.16$). The difference in average thickness of the invasive melanomas in the three groups was highly significant ($p = 0.001$), whereas the difference between the occurrence of melanomas *in situ* in the three groups was of borderline significance ($p = 0.07$).

We do conclude that screening leads to the detection at an earlier age of more melanomas *in situ* and less invasive melanomas. We consider this to be an indication of the effectiveness of our screening program.

TABLE 3
Developmental Stage of Melanomas Detected before the Start of the Screening Program (A), at Initial Examination (B), and during Follow-up Studies (C)

	A	B	C
Total number	21	12	24
Average age at diagnosis (years)	47.1	41.1	28.9
Range (years)	18—87	17—62	16—39
Melanoma *in situ*	1	3	8
Invasive melanoma	20	9	16
Average thickness (mm)[a]	1.88	0.81	0.51
Range (mm)	0.45—4.55	0.30—2.74	0.15—1.01

E. CONSIDERATION OF PEDIGREE VDB (FIGURE 3)

As a comprehensive monograph allows an author to go into some detail, we feel it is instructive to discuss a FAMMM pedigree in which several situations occur that are difficult to interpret or that are even inconclusive, as was the case with Family VDB, originating from a fishing village near Leiden. Family VDB includes two main branches A and B, each consisting of three generations, connected in a preceeding generation by two brothers. Both branches had a separate proband.

Generation III (branch A) consisted of nine sibs, two of whom were already dead at the time of the investigation (III-7 death due to a cerebral hemorrhage at the age of 50; III-12 death due to a pathologically verified sarcoma of the brain at the age of 29); whereas one female member (III-15) refused investigation (in pedigree 2 she had been shown erroneously as being investigated).

We regard individuals III-9, III-16, and III-20 as unaffected, also in view of their unaffected children (n = 8). The father of the proband (III-10) definitely has the FAMMM syndrome, having pathologically verified moles and 3 (out of 5) affected offspring. Individuals III-13 and III-19 might both be considered as obligate gene carriers: III-19 has three out of six children with dysplastic nevi. However, III-13 forms somewhat of a problem: he has five children who were all personally investigated by us; no one showed any recognizable manifestation of the FAMMM syndrome. However, dysplastic nevi did occur in one of his two grandchildren (V-80, aged 13). The mother of this grandchild seemed normal too and is not known to be a member of a family with the FAMMM syndrome, although her family comes from the same village. Since the chance of finding nonpenetrance both in a parent and a grandparent of an affected child seems quite small, we finally regarded individual III-13 as only 50% at risk and his 5 children as 25% at risk, all being unaffected in view of their normal phenotype. As a consequence one might consider the occurrence of dysplastic nevi in V-80 as a "sporadic" event; this is the reason why we did not include her in the analysis. Phenocopies (= sporadic type of DNS) occur in about 10% of the general population, although detailed family studies are usually lacking.

Generation III (branch B) includes nine sibs, four of whom had died before the beginning of the study (III-22 from a carcinoma of the lung at age 65, III-25, and III-28 from cardiovascular disease at the ages of 67 and 32, and III-30 from a cholangiocarcinoma at age 48). Individuals III-31 and III-38 and their 6 children did not show any signs of the FAMMM syndrome and therefore were regarded as normal. Subject III-36 has been regarded as normal too, lacking dysplastic nevi, although we only investigated one of her three children.

Subject III-26 did not show dysplastic nevi, nor did his wife (III-27). Two of their three children were affected: IV-63 had pathologically verified dysplastic moles, while IV-64 had pathologically verified dysplastic moles and a cutaneous melanoma. The spouse (III-27) was a member of a FAMMM family, although she did not show dysplastic moles herself. In this situation it was impossible to find out which one of these partners was a gene carrier. In the analysis, this branch of the family had not been included either.

Subjects III-28 and III-34 must have been obligate gene carriers: III-28 had one affected child (IV-67) and one obligate gene carrier (IV-68) among his 4 children; III-34 had one affected child (IV-74) with one affected grandchild, both living in Australia. The diagnosis in these two has not been verified by us, but according to the family they are being seen at regular intervals by dermatologists and several nevi have been removed.

In conclusion, this pedigree includes three living (+ 1 deceased) melanoma patients (two of which were the probands), 12 (+ 1; V-80) persons having dysplastic nevi, four living (+ 2 possible: III-13 and IV-46) gene carriers (only one of whom (IV-10) has manifest dysplastic nevi himself), and three deceased obligate gene carriers (III-22, III-25, and III-28) on whom we have no information regarding the presence of dysplastic nevi.

Notwithstanding the apparent low penetrance of the gene in the living individuals of generation III (1 out of 4 or 1 out of 5 if III-13 is included), the segregation ratio of the gene in this generation was as expected for a dominant gene. Of the 18 persons, 1 was not investigated and 3 deceased individuals had no children; of the remaining 14 persons, 7 were definite gene carriers. Of the 24 children of these 7 persons, 1 was not investigated; 13 were affected (including the two index cases); and 1 (IV-68) was a nonpenetrant proven gene carrier. The presence of at least four proven nonpenetrant gene carriers in this very well-studied pedigree reveals the hazards of linkage studies in families with the FAMMM syndrome.

III. SUMMARY

Clinical and genetic studies were performed in ten large Dutch families in which a minimum of three individuals with melanomas occurred in at least two consecutive generations. Eight of the families seem to be clustered in two small villages in the neighborhood of Leiden. The inhabitants of these villages have tight religious bonds and even those born after 1950 usually do not move to other parts of the country.

The segregation ratio in these families is not markedly different from 0.5; a minimal rate of nonpenetrance of about 0.16 is included. In these families linkage studies excluded the FAMMM gene to be located on the short arm of chromosome 1. The spectrum of clinical signs characterizing the FAMMM phenotype ranged from an apparent lack of expression (nonpenetrance) through minimal to obvious manifestations. After a follow-up period of 5 years we were able to substantiate the impact of screening these families by a significant decease in the mean Breslow thickness of melanomas diagnosed before the start of the family screening and those diagnosed during follow-up.

REFERENCES

1. **Bergman, W., Palan, A., and Went, L. N.,** Clinical and genetic studies in six Dutch kindreds with the dysplastic nevus syndrome, *Ann. Hum. Genet.*, 50, 249, 1986.
2. **Lynch, H. T., Fusaro, R. M., Kimberling, W. J., Lynch, J. F., and Shannon Danes, B.,** Familial atypical multiple mole melanoma (FAMMM) syndrome: segregation analysis, *J. Med. Genet.*, 20, 342, 1983.
3. **Greene, M. H., Goldin, L. R., Clark, W. H., et al.,** Familial cutaneous malignant melanoma: autosomal dominant trait possibly linked to the Rh locus, *Proc. Nat. Acad. Sci.*, 80, 6071, 1983.
4. **Bale, S. J., Greene, M. H., Murray, C., Goldin, L. R., Johnson, A. H., and Mann, D.,** Hereditary malignant melanoma is not linked to the HLA complex on chromosome 6, *Int. J. Cancer*, 36, 439, 1985.

5. **Happle, R. and Traupe, H.,** Polygene Vererbung der familiairen malignen Melanome, *Hautarzt,* 33, 106, 1982.
6. **Happle, R., Traupe, H., Vakilzadeh, F., and Macher, E.,** Arguments in favor of a polygenic inheritance of precursor nevi, *J. Am. Acad. Dermatol.*, 540, 1982.
7. **Traupe, H., Macher, E., Hamm, H., and Happle, R.,** Mutation rate estimates are not compatible with autosomal dominant inheritance of the dysplastic nevus 'syndrome', *Am. J. Med. Genet.*, 32, 155, 1989.
8. **Bale, S. J., Dracopoli, N. C., Tucker, M. A., Clark, W. H., Fraser, M. C., Stanger, B. Z., et al.,** Mapping the gene for hereditary cutaneous malignant melanoma-dysplastic nevus to chromosome 1*p*, *N. Engl. J. Med.*, 320, 1367, 1989.
9. **van Haeringen, A., Bergman, W., Nelen, M. R., van der Kooy-Meis, E., Hendrikse, I., Wijnen, J. T., et al.,** Exclusion of DNS locus from the short arm of chromosome 1 by linkage studies in Dutch families, *Genomics,* 5, 365, 1989.
10. **Vasen, H. F. A., Bergman, W., van Haeringen, A., Scheffer, E., and van Slooten, E. A.,** The familial dysplastic nevus syndrome. Natural history and the impact of screening on prognosis. A study of nine families in the Netherlands, *Eur. J. Cancer Clin. Oncol.*, 25, 337, 1989.

Chapter 4

OCULAR MELANOMA ASSOCIATED WITH THE FAMILIAL ATYPICAL MULTIPLE MOLE MELANOMA (FAMMM) SYNDROME

Jendo A. Oosterhuis, Loe N. Went, and Wilma Bergman

TABLE OF CONTENTS

I. INTRODUCTION

Melanomas of the uvea and of the skin may be rather similar in histologic appearance but show distinct differences in epidemiological and immunohistologic aspects.

The annual incidence of primary ocular melanoma in Caucasians in 1975 was 1:100,000, and of cutaneous melanomas, 4:100,000.[7] Since then the incidence of cutaneous melanoma has increased considerably, to about 7:100,000 in the Netherlands, but the incidence of uveal melanoma has not increased.

The frequency of the hereditary form of melanoma of the skin has been reported to lie between 0.4 and 12% of all melanomas depending on the intensity and mode of search.[14] When intensive case finding was employed, 10.7% of 666 cutaneous melanoma patients had a positive family history.[41,48] In this book in the chapter on the FAMMM syndrome in the Netherlands, based only on family information, 9.7% were found to have other melanoma patients in the family.

Reports on familial occurrence of intraocular melanomas, on the other hand, have been rather rare, as there are only 15 documented instances reported in literature. The cases have involved siblings in four pedigrees,[25,34,35] two generations in seven pedigrees,[6,18,25,30,41,42,47] and three generations in four pedigrees.[8,13,25,49] In the few reported instances of familial intraocular melanoma the lesions tend to follow autosomal dominant mode of inheritance.[25]

There is also a difference regarding the development of multiple melanomas. Multiple primary cutaneous melanomas are reported to occur in 19% of patients with a family history of melanoma and in 1 to 4% of the nonfamilial cases.[22] In the eye, development of multiple primary melanomas is uncommon because only eight patients with multiple separate melanomas of the choroid in one eye have been described.[46] Melanomas fortunately tend to develop in one eye only and rarely occur in the other eye as well. Only 23 cases of a bilateral uveal melanoma have been reported.[12,24,32,46] Jensen[20] had no bilateral cases among his 295 melanoma patients; we have observed only one case in more than 300 patients.

In immunohistologic respect there is a difference between ocular and cutaneous melanoma.[44] Twenty-five uveal melanomas were stained with seven monoclonal antibodies recognizing different antigens for cutaneous melanomas. Expression of antigens for uveal melanomas differed markedly from that for primary cutaneous melanomas.

II. REVIEW OF PATIENTS WITH OCULAR MELANOMA ASSOCIATED WITH CUTANEOUS DYSPLASTIC NEVI

In the literature only six patients have been described harboring an ocular melanoma — five with a uveal melanoma and one with a conjunctival melanoma — associated with cutaneous melanoma and/or dysplastic nevi (atypical multiple moles). Only in three of them did family information give evidence of the presence of the FAMMM syndrome. A seventh patient had a dysplastic nevus of the conjunctiva and cutaneous dysplastic nevi with familial evidence of the presence of the FAMMM syndrome.

Bellet et al.[5] reported on a spindle B cell melanoma of ciliary body and choroid observed in a 54-year-old male. About 1 year after enucleation cutaneous examination revealed numerous scattered pigmented lesions. Histologic examination of biopsy specimens disclosed the presence of dysplastic nevi. Superficial spreading melanoma was the histologic diagnosis of a pigmented lesion on the right scapula. This report did not provide data on the family of the patient.

Abramson et al.[1] described a 51-year-old male with a large tumor located in the iris and ciliary body of his right eye which had been treated by iridocyclectomy. Histopathologic examination showed spindle B and epitheloid melanoma cells. General medical examination at that time revealed multiple pigmented lesions in the skin of the upper part of the patient's back. Two suspicious moles were biopsied; both were diagnosed as malignant melanoma associated with atypical multiple moles, named by Abramson B-K moles. No data on the patient's family were available.

Results of two families have been published by Greene et al.[15] In the first family a 56-year-old female had her left eye, which contained a large tumor, enucleated. Histopathologic examination revealed a spindle B cell uveal melanoma with spindle cell hyperplasia at its periphery, suggestive of a precursor nevus. Careful dermatologic examination disclosed a normal mole pattern without evidence of the presence of the FAMMM syndrome. Five moles were removed from the 27-year-old daughter of the patient. Four years later a biopsy of a recurrent skin pigmentation disclosed a cutaneous melanoma. Histologic examination of a mole removed at the same time and review of the previously removed moles revealed melanocytic dysplasia of the type that occurs in the FAMMM syndrome.

In the second family, a 60-year-old man developed an intraocular tumor which was treated by enucleation. Histopathology showed a spindle B cell and epithelioid cell choroidal melanoma with an adjacent small focus of choroidal spindle cells suggestive of a choroidal nevus. One of his two daughters noticed several changing moles at the age of 55, which on histologic examination were classified as microinvasive lentigo malignant melanoma. A recurrent pigmentation excised 5 years later was again classified as lentigo malignant melanoma. Clinically, this patient had in addition many dysplastic nevi, but further biopsies have not been performed.

Albert et al.[2] reported on the eye of a 75-year-old man which was enucleated because it harbored a choroidal melanoma. Histopathology revealed a large tumor with predominantly spindle B cells. Dermatologic examination for melanocytic lesions was negative. The son of the patient had a cutaneous melanoma which was removed at the age of 41. Biopsies of several pigmented lesions showed compound nevi with dysplastic-appearing melanocytes. Two grandchildren have clinically mildly atypical melanocytic lesions. These findings are strongly indicative of the presence of the FAMMM syndrome.

Association of dysplastic nevi with melanoma or atypical conjunctival lesions has only been described in two patients. Friedman et al.[10] described a 29-year-old female who, on dermatologic examination, showed multiple nevi with clinical features of dysplastic nevi; a biopsy confirmed the diagnosis. Ten years prior to this a salmon-colored pigmented lesion had been removed from the left conjunctiva. Review of the section revealed a conjunctival malignant melanoma.

Jakobiec et al.[19] examined a 37-year-old female with cutaneous dysplastic nevi and a dysplastic conjunctival nevus which they felt had been intercepted in its trajectory towards melanoma. A sister of this patient had a cutaneous melanoma removed.

Apart from the aforementioned cases there has been a rather bizarre case history of an Algerian boy who already at the age of 3 months had complaints caused by an intraocular melanoma.[21] Scattered pink or light brown spots on the skin changed into black indolent, firm elements of 1 to 5 mm in diameter. Biopsy showed a typical compound nevus with some features of dysplastic nevi. Jensen et al.[21] considered this to be a sporadic case of the FAMMM syndrome. In our experience, however, recognition — let alone change — of dysplastic nevi never occurred at that age.

III. REVIEW OF PATIENTS WITH UVEAL AND CUTANEOUS MELANOMA APPARENTLY WITHOUT CUTANEOUS DYSPLASTIC NEVI

There is a rather limited number of nine possibly ten reports on patients in whom cutaneous and ocular melanomas occurred as double primary malignancies or with two types of melanoma in different members of the same family; in none of these cases has the FAMMM syndrome been mentioned by the authors.

The first case of simultaneous occurrence of primary melanoma of the eye and the skin has been reported by Paton and Thomas[33] but doubts have been raised regarding the malignancy of the choroidal tumor.

A 72-year-old woman had a primary melanoma of the periorbital skin on her right side, primary acquired melanosis of the conjunctiva, and a pigmented tumor of the choroid. Clinically, the latter showed the characteristics of a benign choroidal nevus: it was 2 mm in diameter and 0.3 mm in thickness and had not produced a visual field defect. Although histology of the choroidal tumor was reported to reveal a melanoma, a review by Bellet et al.,[5] of the published micrographs, suggested that the tumor would be classified as a choroidal nevus according to histologic criteria of MacLean et al.[29] However, apart from spindle A cells which comprised the bulk of the tumor, spindle B cells also were found. It is of interest that the patient's brother had his right eye enucleated 9 years previously because of the presence of a malignant choroidal melanoma.

The case history described by Turkington[43] concerns a male who at the age of 31 had his left eye enucleated for malignant melanoma. Several years prior to his death, at the age of 63, he had developed multiple subcutaneous tumor nodules over most areas of his body; biopsies revealed melanoma of the skin and abdomen. The patient's sister noticed at the age of 40 enlargement of a black mole on her forehead; about six months later she died from gastric and cerebral melanoma metastasis. A maternal uncle and a paternal granduncle of these patients had died with widespread skin and cerebral melanoma metastases.

In an addendum to an article Lynch et al.[25] provided information on data of two families referred to them by an ophthalmologist. A man in one family had an intraocular malignant melanoma, while his son had cutaneous malignant melanoma. In the other family a woman had an intraocular malignant melanoma of her left eye, while her sister had two toes removed as a consequence of cutaneous malignant melanoma. All tumors were histologically verified.

Lynch and Krush[25] reported on a 61-year-old female with an intraocular melanoma while her sister at age 51 had a cutaneous melanoma. In another family a 74-year-old male had an intraocular melanoma; his son at age 44 had a cutaneous melanoma. All four tumors were histologically confirmed.

In a male patient described by Grimstvedt,[17] and quoted by Greene et al.,[15] an intraocular melanoma was found at the age of 51. His mother, two of his daughters, and one son were found to have a cutaneous melanoma at the age of 45, 49, 40 and 47 years, respectively.

Augsburger et al.[4] described the findings of a diffuse primary malignant melanoma of the uvea, mixed cell type, in a 64-year-old male who died 9 months later presumably from a metastatic malignant tumor of the liver. Eleven years previously a cutaneous melanoma of his lower lip had been excised, followed by neck dissection for lymph node metastasis.

Korting[23] reported on a 32-year-old male who had his right eye enucleated which contained a choroidal melanoma. Nine years later a cutaneous melanoma was removed from his chest.

Weber[50] et al. described a 48-year-old male with visual complaints caused by a choroidal melanoma of 9 mm in diameter and 3 mm in elevation. Histopathology revealed a spindle type melanoma probably originating from a choroidal nevus. Dermatologic examination performed at the same time disclosed a cutaneous melanoma of the right ear among multiple benign lentigines: the melanoma was histologically confirmed.

IV. OWN MATERIAL

Our own material consists of seven families with ocular melanoma associated with cutaneous dysplastic nevi or melanoma; in all families the FAMMM syndrome also was found. Data on the first two families have been published previously.[28,30] Family members were examined in the Departments of Ophthalmology and Dermatology of Leiden University

Hospital. The results on the other five families (cases 3 to 7) are being published in a separate paper.[45]

V. CASE REPORTS

A. CASE 1

A 57-year-old man was referred to our clinic in May 1978 for evaluation of an intraocular mass in his right eye. His medical history revealed that a tumor with a small satellite lesion had been removed from the scalp at the age of 53; this lesion proved to be a melanoma. At the age of 54 a melanoma was excised from the skin of his right shoulder and another from the gluteal region.

On admission, visual acuity was 1/60 for the right eye and 6/6 for the left eye. Ophthalmoscopy revealed an elevated, darkly pigmented, solid choroidal mass arising from the temporal equatorial region in the right eye. It measured approximately 13 mm in diameter and 8 mm in elevation. At that time the ocular media of the left eye were clear, and on ophthalmoscopy no abnormalities were observed in this eye. Fluorescein angiography showed an early mottled fluorescence and late diffuse staining of the tumor. A 48-hour 32P uptake test was strongly positive, +389%, which is far above the critical level of +60%. A thorough medical examination for metastatic disease, which included chest X-ray, liver function studies, and a liver scintigram, was negative. The clinical diagnosis was melanoma of the choroid. Histologic examination after enucleation confirmed that the tumor was a melanoma of the epithelioid cell type which had already invaded halfway into the sclera.

Eight months after enucleation of the right eye the patient complained of blurred vision of his left eye. Within one day the corrected visual acuity dropped from 6/6 to 5/60. Ophthalmoscopy revealed a rapidly spreading retinal detachment, becoming subtotal. At the lower periphery, a tumor with a diameter of 10 mm, an elevation of 8 mm, and relatively little pigment was visible. Ultrasonography and a positive 32P uptake test of +181% supported the clinical diagnosis of melanoma of the choroid. After enucleation, the histologic examination confirmed the diagnosis. The tumor contained mainly epithelioid cells which had penetrated through Bruch's membrane but had not invaded the sclera. The extensive medical examination was repeated. This time the chest X-ray tomogram showed 3 lesions indicative of metastases.

In subsequent months the general condition gradually deteriorated owing to metastatic spreading. Nine months after enucleation of the second eye the patient died.

This patient was a member of a family in which the FAMMM syndrome occurred and which has been studied extensively; in the publication of Lynch et al.,[28] he is III-8; in the pedigree in the publication of Lynch et al.,[27] he appears as an unaffected individual as IV-16 of pedigree 2.

B. CASE 2

A 52-year-old man was referred because of a 4 D prominent tumor of his left eye with the aspect of a choroidal melanoma, measuring 5 mm in diameter and located superior to the posterior pole. Corrected visual acuity was 0.6. Fluorescein angiography showed a pattern typical of choroidal melanoma: perimetry revealed an absolute scotoma at the site of the tumor. The 48-hour 32P uptake test was positive, +107%. In view of the clinical diagnosis of melanoma of the choroid, the eye was enucleated. On histologic examination the tumor proved to be a spindle B cell melanoma of the choroid.

The medical history was significant in that a pigmented skin lesion on his arm had been excised 2 years previously. Examination in the Department of Dermatology revealed a pigmented spot at the margin of the scar resulting from the previous removal. After excision, histologic examination showed the tumor to be a cutaneous melanoma. Two pigmented lesions were excised from the skin of the back; on histologic examination they proved to be benign nevi. Thirteen years later the patient was still in good health.

Dermatologic examination of the daughter, the only child of the patient, revealed the presence of multiple dysplastic nevi, thus establishing the diagnosis of the FAMMM syndrome.

C. CASE 3

A 16-year-old female had a pigmented lesion removed from the conjunctiva of her left eye. One and a half years later she was operated on again for a recurrence of the pigmented lesion of the conjunctiva and cornea. The histopathologic diagnosis of the primary lesion was a conjunctival nevus and of the recurrence, a conjunctival melanoma. The skin showed multiple moles with dysplastic characteristics, confirmed by biopsy. The diagnosis of the FAMMM syndrome was established by the presence of multiple dysplastic nevi in her sister and father. This is the second case of a conjunctival melanoma associated with the FAMMM syndrome; the first case, which we have discussed earlier, has been published by Friedman et al.[10]

D. CASE 4

A 20-year-old man had his left eye enucleated because of choroidal melanoma. Two years later dermatologic examination revealed multiple moles, scattered over his body. They were clinically very characteristic of dysplastic nevi. The presence of the FAMMM syndrome was clinically proven by the presence of multiple dysplastic nevi in the patient's two brothers and his mother.

E. CASE 5

This patient was a woman who at the age of 51 had a cutaneous melanoma removed from her left elbow. Seventeen years later, at the age of 68, her left eye was enucleated because of a large, mushroom-shaped choroidal melanoma which on histopathology contained partly spindle cells and partly epithelioid cells. It was established that the choroidal melanoma was a primary melanoma and not a metastatic neoplasm. Examination in the Department of Dermatology showed clear signs of dysplastic nevi in a daughter and a son of the patient, thus establishing the presence of the FAMMM syndrome.

F. CASE 6

A 71-year-old woman, examined because of visual loss of her right eye, showed, aside from a cataract, a bluish subconjunctival discoloration superior to the cornea and a brownish solid mass in the superior part of the anterior chamber. Histopathologic examination after enucleation revealed a large melanoma of the ciliary body with extension into the chamber angle and extrascleral outgrowth. One of her daughters had died from a melanoma of the skin of the sole of her foot. Two other daughters and two sons of her still-living ten children had clinically dysplastic nevi, thus establishing the diagnosis of the FAMMM syndrome.

G. CASE 7

The proband was a 33-year-old female. She had a cutaneous melanoma (Clark III Breslow 1.0 mm) on her breast during her first pregnancy. She also had many large atypical nevi, several of which were excised and found to be dysplastic on histologic examination. The proband's only sister is reported to have many moles as well. Her father had a pigmented lesion removed from the conjunctiva of his right lower eyelid at the age of 53. This lesion had been there for several years and turned out to be a conjunctival melanoma. Three years later a small pigmented lesion was noticed on the conjunctiva of his upper eyelid again on the right side. On removal this proved to be a second conjunctival melanoma, which, according to the pathologist, probably originated from acquired melanosis.

VI. DISCUSSION

Opinions are controversial regarding the existence of a causative relationship between cutaneous melanoma and ocular melanoma. Is the link between the two pigment cell malignancies the FAMMM syndrome? Do patients with cutaneous melanoma or dysplastic nevi in families with the FAMMM syndrome have an increased risk of developing an intraocular melanoma? Or should the association between the FAMMM syndrome and the intraocular melanoma be seen as a coincidental finding?

In the reports on familial occurrence of intraocular melanoma, unfortunately information on the possible presence of the FAMMM syndrome in these families is lacking.

Histopathologic studies of dysplastic nevi of the skin have been reported extensively. Whereas the biopsy of a suspicious nevus of the skin is a simple procedure for a dermatologist, biopsy of nevi of iris and choroid is for technical and ethical reasons not permissible. Such nevi are only found accidentally, sometimes in eyes enucleated for treatment of uveal melanoma. Thus, only clinical studies can provide information on the prevalence of ocular nevi in patients with cutaneous melanoma.

Albert et al.[3] found patients with cutaneous melanoma to have a significantly higher frequency (51%) of iris nevi as compared to control subjects (39%); for choroidal nevi the frequency was 4% and 1%, respectively; but the numbers were too small for statistical evaluation.

Rodriguez-Sains[39] performed a similar study in 92 patients with dysplastic nevi. A significantly higher percentage was found in these patients vs. controls: for conjunctival nevi 9.8% vs. 1.8%, for iris nevi 31.5% vs. 13.0%, and for choroidal nevi 18.5% vs. 4.6%.

In an extended study Rodriguez-Sains[40] reported on 257 patients with biopsy-proven dysplastic nevi. As compared to 264 controls they showed a significantly higher percentage of conjunctival nevi 8.6% vs. 1.1%, iris nevi 24.9% vs. 9.5%, and choroidal nevi, 14.4% vs. 5.3%, as well as a statistically significant greater number of iris nevi per patient.

Based on these findings of a relationship between dysplastic nevi of the skin and ocular nevi and knowing that an association exists between dysplastic nevi and melanoma of the skin, Rodriguez-Sains[36,38,39] suggested that an association might exist as well between ocular and cutaneous melanoma in families in which the FAMMM syndrome does occur. He believes therefore that regular indirect ophthalmoscopical examination should be performed in patients with the dysplastic nevus syndrome.

Greene et al.[15] disagreed with this approach and advocated ocular examination only as part of a general physical examination. In their study of 26 patients with hereditary cutaneous melanoma and/or the dysplastic nevus syndrome, thorough ophthalmologic examination failed to show intraocular melanoma or atypical choroidal nevi. Furthermore they did not find cases of intraocular melanoma in their cohort of 14 families in which the dysplastic nevus syndrome occurred and thus concluded that the occasional reports of such a combination were due to chance. However, in view of the limited number of patients studied, they did not rule out the possibility that larger surveys might show a relationship between nevi and choroidal melanoma.

We feel, however, that such a combination is based on a causal relationship: we conclude this from our findings in the seven patients described in this chapter; the FAMMM syndrome has been established in all their families. They were all observed within a period of 10 years. In one of these patients (nr 1) five primary melanomas developed within a period of 4 years: three cutaneous melanomas (scalp, shoulder, and gluteal region), and a choroidal melanoma first in the right eye and 8 months later in the left eye. This cannot be considered as a coincidental association.

Our number of seven patients, all from one university center, exceeded the number of six patients with ocular melanoma associated with cutaneous melanoma and/or dysplastic nevi hitherto described in the literature. We have analyzed the publications on these six patients in the first part of this chapter and found that in only three of them, limited family studies, provided evidence of the presence of the FAMMM syndrome. The apparent concentration of cases around Leiden, which seems to be at variance with the great rarity of publications concerning the subject, can be explained by the collaborative efforts of the departments of dermatology, ophthalmology, and human genetics of the medical faculty in Leiden. Thus, we are convinced that many more — as yet undetected — instances of ocular melanoma actually find their origin in families in which the FAMMM syndrome does occur. To discover these, a careful dermatologic analysis of the skin will be required, not only of patients with ocular melanoma but also of their parents, sibs, and children, since there are many instances of nonpenetrance of the genes responsible for the FAMMM syndrome (see Chapter 3). Anamnestic information from the patients and their family members is in this respect quite insufficient.

Our conclusion from the foregoing is therefore that the gene responsible for the FAMMM syndrome does not only lead to a markedly increased risk for the development of cutaneous melanoma, but also may occasionally lead to the development of an ocular melanoma, perhaps originating from an ocular nevus.[39] To give a quantitative assessment of the chances for such an occurrence seems hazardous; this is obvious from the discussions on this subject between Rodriguez-Sains,[37-39] Greene et al.,[15,16] Fusaro et al.,[11] and Albert et al.[2]

However, it is important to realize that early detection of a choroidal melanoma when its dimensions are still small, makes the tumor amenable for conservative treatment such as radiotherapy.[31] This may destroy the tumor, with conservation of the eye and eyesight.

We agree with the suggestion of Folberg,[9] that the ophthalmologic screening could be carried out according to the advice of the American Academy of Ophthalmology. It recommends that individuals have occasional ocular examinations from puberty to the age of 40 to detect asymptomatic conditions, and that an ophthalmic evaluation be performed every 2 to 4 years after the age of 40.

REFERENCES

1. **Abramson, D. H., Rodriguez-Sains, R. S., and Rubman, R.,** B-K Mole syndrome, cutaneous and ocular malignant melanoma, *Arch. Ophthalmol.*, 98, 1397, 1980.
2. **Albert, D. M., Chang, M. A., Lamping, K., Weiter, J., and Sober, A.,** The dysplastic nevus syndrome, a pedigree with primary malignant melanomas of the choroid and skin, *Ophthalmology,* 92, 1728, 1985.
3. **Albert, D. M., Searl, S. S., Forget, B., Lavin, P. T., Kirkwood, J., and Nordlund, J. J.,** Uveal findings in patients with cutaneous melanoma, *Am. J. Ophthalmol.*, 95, 474, 1983.
4. **Augsburger, J. J., Shields, J. A., Mastrangelo, M. J., and Frank, P. E.,** Diffuse primary malignant melanoma after prior primary cutaneous malignant melanoma, *Arch. Ophthalmol.*, 98, 1261, 1980.
5. **Bellet, R. E., Shields, J. A., Soll, D. B., and Bernardino, E. A.,** Primary choroidal and cutaneous melanomas occurring in a patient with the B-K mole syndrome phenotype, *Am. J. Ophthalmol.*, 89, 567, 1980.
6. **Bowen, S. F., Brady, H., and Jones, V. L.,** Malignant melanoma of the eye occurring in two successive generations, *Arch. Ophthalmol.*, 71, 805, 1964.
7. **Cutler, S. J. and Young, J. L.,** Third National Cancer Survey, Incidence Data, *Natl. Cancer Inst. Monog.* No. 41, U.S. Government Printing Office, Washington, D.C., 1975.
8. **Davenport, R. C.,** Family history of choroidal sarcoma, *Br. J. Ophthalmol.*, 11, 443, 1927.
9. **Folberg, R.,** Letter to the editor, *Am. J. Ophthalmol.*, 96, 815, 1983.
10. **Friedman, R. J., Rodriguez-Sains, R., and Jakobiec, F.,** Ophthalmologic oncology; conjunctival malignant melanoma in association with sporadic dysplastic nevus syndrome, *Dermatol. Surg. Oncol.*, 13, 31, 1987.
11. **Fusaro, R. M., Lynch, H. T., Oosterhuis, J. A., and Went, L. N.,** The familial occurrence of cutaneous melanoma and the dysplastic nevus syndrome, *Am. J. Ophthalmol.*, 97, 802, 1984.

12. **Gragoudas, E. S., Goitein, M., Verhey, L., Munzenreider, J., Suits, H. D., and Koehler, A.,** Proton beam irradiation, an alternative to enucleation for intraocular melanomas, *Ophthalmology,* 87, 571, 1980.
13. **Green, G. J., Hong, W. K., Everett, J. R., Bhutani, R., and Amick, R. M.,** Familial intraocular malignant melanoma, a case report, *Cancer,* 41, 2481, 1978.
14. **Greene, M. H. and Fraumeni, Jr., J. F.,** The hereditary variant of malignant melanoma, in Clark, W. H., Goldman, L., and Mastrangelo, M. J., *Human Malignant Melanoma,* Grune & Stratton, New York, 1979, 139.
15. **Greene, M. H., Sanders, R. J., Chu, F. C., Clark, Jr., W. H., Elder, D. E., and Cogan, D. G.,** The familial occurrence of cutaneous melanoma, intraocular melanoma, and the dysplastic nevus syndrome, *Am. J. Ophthalmol.,* 96, 238, 1983.
16. **Greene, M. H., Sanders, R. J., Chu, F. C., Clark, W. H., Elder, D. E., and Cogan, D. G.,** Letter to the editor, *Am. J. Ophthalmol.,* 97, 115, 1984.
17. **Grimstvedt, A. M.,** Familiaer forekomst av maligne melanomer, *Tidsskr. Nor. Laegeforen.,* 89, 1900, 1969.
18. **Gutmann, G.,** Casuistischer Beitrag zur Lehre von den Geschwulsten des Augapfels, *Arch. Augenheilk.,* 31, 158, 1895.
19. **Jakobiec, F. A., Zuckerman, B. D., Berlin, A. J., Odell, P., MacRae, D. W., and Tuthill, R. J.,** Unusual melanocytic nevi of the conjunctiva, *Am. J. Ophthalmol.,* 100, 100, 1985.
20. **Jensen, O. A.,** Malignant melanomas of the uvea in Denmark, 1943—1952, a clinical, histopathological, and prognostic study, *Acta Ophthalmol. Suppl.,* 75, 76, 1963.
21. **Jensen, O. A., Movin, M., and Müller, J.,** Malignant melanoma of the choroid in an infant with the dysplastic naevus syndrome, *Acta Ophthalmol.,* 65, 91, 1987.
22. **Kopf, A. W., Bart, R. S., and Rodriguez-Sains, R. S.,** Malignant melanoma, a review, *J. Dermatol. Surg. Oncol.,* 3, 41, 1977.
23. **Korting, H. C.,** Coincidence of superficial spreading melanoma of the skin and fusiform melanoma of the eye in a Caucasian male, *XVI Congress Int. Dermatol.,* Tokyo, May 23—28, 1982, University of Tokyo Press, 1982, 221.
24. **Lommatzsch, P. K., Hallermann, D., and von Domarus, D.,** Treatment of bilateral choroidal malignant melanoma, *Dev. Ophthalmol.,* 2, 105, 1981.
25. **Lynch, H. T., Anderson, D. E., and Krush, A. J.,** Heredity and intraocular malignant melanoma, study of two families and review of forty-five cases, *Cancer,* 21, 119, 1968.
26. **Lynch, H. T. and Krush, A. J.,** Heredity and malignant melanoma, implications for early cancer detection, *Can. Med. Assoc. J.,* 99, 17, 1968.
27. **Lynch, H. T., Frichot, B. C., Lynch, P., Lynch, J., and Guirgis, H. A.,** Family studies of malignant melanoma and associated cancer, *Surg. Gynecol. Obstet.,* 141, 517, 1975.
28. **Lynch, H. T., Fusaro, R. M., Pester, J., Oosterhuis, J. A., Went, L. N., Rumke, P., Neering, H., and Lynch, J. F.,** Tumour spectrum in the FAMMM syndrome, *Br. J. Cancer,* 44, 553, 1981.
29. **MacLean, I. W., Zimmerman, L. E., and Evans, R. M.,** Reappraisal of Callander's spindle A type of malignant melanoma of the choroid and ciliary body, *Am. J. Ophthalmol.,* 86, 557, 1978.
30. **Oosterhuis, J. A., Went, L. N., and Lynch, H. T.,** Primary choroidal and cutaneous melanomas, bilateral choroidal melanomas, and familial occurrence of melanomas, *Br. J. Ophthalmol.,* 66, 230, 1982.
31. **Oosterhuis, J. A.,** Conservative treatment modalities of choroidal melanomas, in *Ophthalmic Tumours,* Oosterhuis, J. A., Ed., Dr. W. Junk Publishers, Dordrecht, 1985, 27.
32. **Osborn, E. L., Walker, J. P., and Weiter, J. J.,** Bilateral choroidal melanomas, a case report, *Ann. Ophthalmol.,* 12, 1154, 1980.
33. **Paton, D. and Thomas, L. B.,** Simultaneous occurrence of primary malignant melanomas of the eye and the skin, *Arch. Ophthalmol.,* 62, 645, 1959.
34. **Pfingst, A. O. and Graves, S.,** Melanosarcoma of choroid occurring in two brothers, *Arch. Ophthalmol.,* 50, 431, 1921.
35. **Reese, A. B.,** *Tumors of the Eye,* Harper & Row, New York, 1963, 219.
36. **Rodriguez-Sains, R. S.,** Are concurrent or subsequent malignant melanomas in the skin and eye related or coincidental?, *J. Dermatol. Surg. Oncol.,* 6, 915, 1980.
37. **Rodriguez-Sains, R. S.,** Letter to the editor, *Am. J. Ophthalmol.,* 96, 257, 1983.
38. **Rodriguez-Sains, R. S.,** Letter to the editor, *Am. J. Ophthalmol.,* 97, 114, 1984.
39. **Rodriguez-Sains, R. S.,** Ocular findings in patients with dysplastic nevus syndrome, *Ophthalmology,* 93, 661, 1986.
40. **Rodriguez-Sains, R. S.,** Ocular findings in patients with dysplastic nevus syndrome, an update, presented at the American Academy of Ophthalmology annual meeting, *Ophthalmology,* in press.
41. **Sutherland, C. M., Kloepfer, H. W., Mansell, P. W. A., et al.,** Familial melanoma, in *Pigment Cell,* Vol. 2, S. Karger, Basel, 1976, 421.
42. **Tasman, W.,** Familial intraocular melanoma, *Trans. Am. Acad. Ophthalmol. Otolaryngol.,* 74, 955, 1970.

43. **Turkington, R. W.,** Familial factor in malignant melanoma, *J. Am. Med. Assoc.*, 192, 77, 1965.
44. **Van der Pol, J. P., Jager, M. J., de Wolff-Rouendaal, Ringens, P. J., Vennegoor, C., and Ruiter, D. J.,** Heterogeneous expression of melanoma-associated antigens in uveal melanomas, *Curr. Eye Res.*, 6, 757, 1987.
45. **Vink, J., Crijns, M. W., Bergman, W., Oosterhuis, J. A., and Went, L. N.,** Ocular melanoma in families with dysplastic nevus syndrome (DNS), *J. Am. Acad. Dermatol.*, 23, 858, 1990.
46. **Völcker, H. E. and Naumann, G. O. H.,** Multicentric primary malignant melanomas of the choroid, *Br. J. Ophthalmol.*, 62, 408, 1978.
47. **Waardenburg, P. J.,** Melanosarcoma van het oog bij verschillende leden eener zelfde familie, *Ned. Tijdschr. Geneesk.*, 84, 4718, 1940.
48. **Wallace, D. C., Beardmore, G. L., and Exton, L. A.,** Familial malignant melanoma, *Ann. Surg.*, 177, 15, 1973.
49. **Walker, J. P., Weiter, J. J., Albert, D. M., Osborn, E. L., and Weichselbaum, R. R.,** Uveal malignant melanoma in three generations of the same family, *Am. J. Ophthalmol.*, 88, 723, 1979.
50. **Weber, F., Harms, H., and Babel, J.,** Mélanomes simultanés de la choroide et de la peau, *J. Franc. Ophthalmol.*, 5, 109, 1982.

Chapter 5

HISTOPATHOLOGICAL CRITERIA REQUIRED FOR THE DIAGNOSIS OF FAMILIAL DYSPLASTIC NEVI

D. J. Ruiter, P. M. Steylen, J. van der Wiel-Miezenbeek, S. C. Henzen-Logmans, W. J. Mooi, W. Bergman, and E. Scheffer

TABLE OF CONTENTS

I. INTRODUCTION

Histopathologic examination of a given pigmented skin lesion in a familial dysplastic nevus patient is required for the following reasons: (1) to confirm the diagnosis of dysplastic nevus (DN), (2) to assess the degree of atypia, and (3) to exclude melanoma. The clinical criteria for selecting a pigmented lesion for diagnostic excision will be discussed elsewhere in this volume.

In order to provide a basis for clinical decisions on treatment and further management of the patient, the histopathologic diagnosis should be reliable. This requires a high level of efficacy of the diagnostic procedure, i.e., of the histopathologic criteria used and of their interpretation.

Since many histopathologic features have been put forward as criteria for the diagnosis of DN,[1-6] we will first discuss the relevant literature. Subsequently we will discuss the methodology of efficacy studies that has been used to evaluate a diagnostic test. In addition we present our data on such an efficacy study performed on DN and discuss their implications. Finally, our experience with the daily use of the histopathologic criteria based on this study will be briefly described.

II. LITERATURE REVIEW ON HISTOPATHOLOGIC FEATURES USED AS DIAGNOSTIC CRITERIA FOR DYSPLASTIC NEVI

We use the term ''dysplastic nevus'' (DN) as synonymous with atypical mole, since it has been generally accepted. For the sake of clarity we now will discuss the terms ''atypia'' and ''dysplasia''. *Atypia* can be defined as a phenotypic deviation from the normal aspect of a cell or tissue. It can be recognized morphologically as a disturbance of the regular appearance of cells or of a tissue, caused by variations in the size and shape of the cells, by enlargement, irregularity, and hyperchromatism of the nuclei, and by disorderly arrangement of the cells within the tissue.[7] Thus, according to this definition, atypia includes both cellular and architectural changes. Some authors use the term dysplasia as a synonym of atypia.[8,9] However, we consider atypia as a *diagnostic feature,* whereas dysplasia is a *histopathologic diagnosis*. Acceptable synonyms for dysplasia in our opinion are *atypical hyperplasia* or *atypical proliferation*.

The histopathological features which have been used as diagnostic criteria for DN can be divided into (1) architectural atypia (see Figure 1), (2) cellular atypia (see Figure 2), and (3) stromal reactions (see Figure 3). It should be noted here that no differences in histopathologic features have been reported between familial and nonfamilial DN lesions.[10,11] Therefore, the features of both types of DN will be discussed. Features of architectural and cellular atypia and stromal reactions based on the literature[1-6] are listed in Table 1 and are alluded to in the following paragraphs.

A. ARCHITECTURAL ATYPIA

Junctional activity has been defined as intraepidermal melanocytic proliferation along the dermoepidermal junction. Melanocytic proliferation may appear in a lentiginous pattern, i.e., as a layer of single cells confined to the basal layer or slightly extending above it; alternatively, proliferation may appear in a nested (nevoid) pattern. Nests may alternate with a lentiginous melanocytic pattern in a single lesion. Junctional activity has been interpreted to be present when the number of melanocytes was increased, either as single cells or as loose aggregates, along several adjacent rete ridges in the lesion. In benign lentigines such as lentigo simplex or lentigo senilis, the melanocytes have a preference for the tips of the rete ridges, as is the case for nests in focal melanocytic proliferations in common nevi.

Rete ridge preference is considered to be absent when solitary units and nests of me-

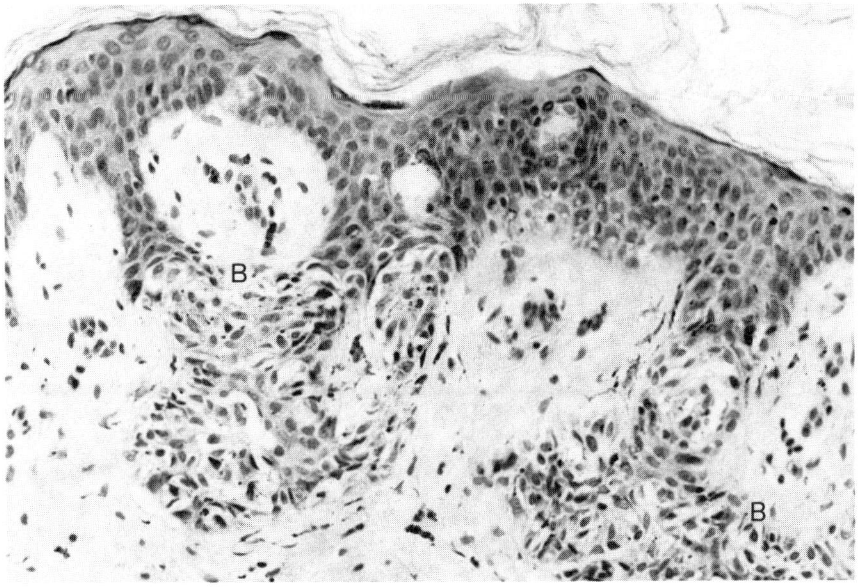

FIGURE 1. Features of architectural atypia in a dysplastic nevus lesion shown here are irregular junctional nests and bridging (B). (Magnification × 160.)

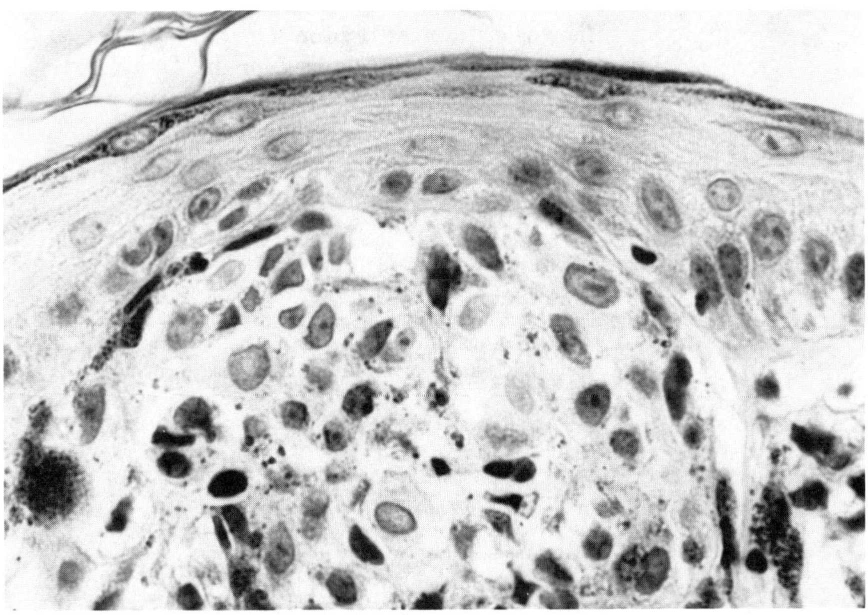

FIGURE 2. Features of cellular atypia in a dysplastic nevus lesion shown here are large prominent melanocytes, large melanocytic nuclei, and nuclear pleomorphism. (Magnification × 400.)

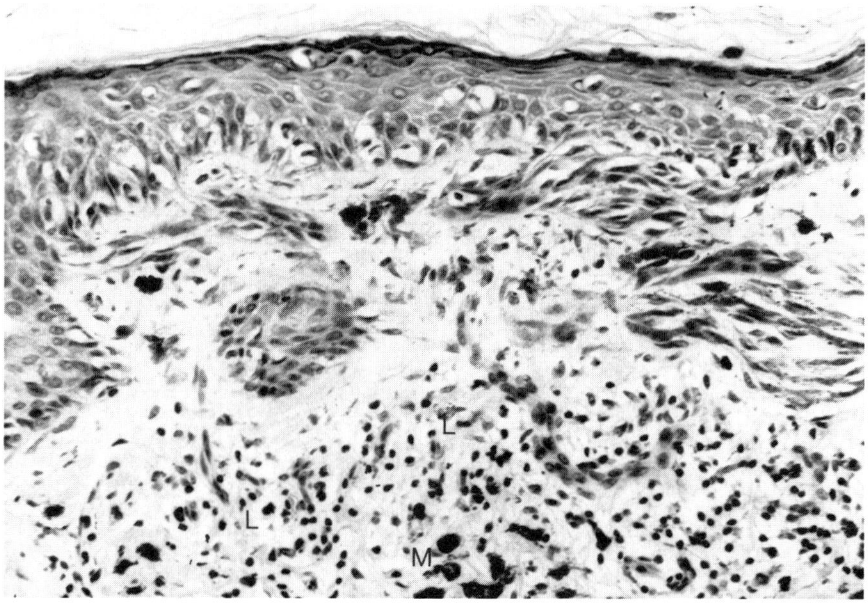

FIGURE 3. Features of stromal reactions in a dysplastic nevus lesion shown here are an aggregate-like lymphocytic infiltrate (L) and accumulation of melanophages (M). (Magnification × 160.)

TABLE 1
Histologic Features Used in the Literature[1-6] as Criteria Required for the Diagnosis of Dysplastic Nevus

Features of Architectural Atypia

Architectural atypia
Increased junctional activity
Loss of melanocytic preference for the rete ridges
Irregularity of the configuration of the rete ridges
Irregularity of junctional nests
Bridging of junctional nests
Impairment of maturation of the dermal component

Features of Cellular Atypia

Large prominent melanocytes
Dusty melanin pigment
Nuclear pleomorphism
Large nuclei
Prominent nucleoli
Prominent retraction artifact

Stromal Reactions

Lymphocytic infiltrate
Fibroplasia
Angioneogenesis
Accumulation of melanophages

lanocytes are arranged at the side of the rete ridges or over the top of dermal papillae. Absence of rete ridge preference can be present locally or throughout the lesion. The presence of elongated, club-shaped, and irregular rete ridges can be observed. Nests have been designated as pleomorphic or irregular when they show considerable variation in size and shape. Bridging is the phenomenon where horizontally oriented nests of melanocytes connect adjacent rete ridges. Impairment of maturation in the deeper parts of the dermal nevocellular component is present when it contains either melanin or relatively large nuclei.

B. CELLULAR ATYPIA

Enlargement and pleomorphism of melanocytes, either solitary or in small nests along the dermoepidermal junction, has been assessed by comparing them to the size of melanocytes in the adjacent normal skin. Dust-like melanin pigment in the cytoplasm of melanocytes can be present. Nuclear pleomorphism has been considered to be present when melanocytic nuclei showed a greater variation in size and shape than those in adjacent normal skin. Large melanocytic nuclei and prominent nucleoli have been observed, but not further defined. The presence of prominent melanocytic retraction artifacts has been noted.

C. STROMAL REACTIONS

The presence and distribution of lymphocytic infiltrate in the dermis has been observed. Increase of fibroblasts and accumulation of collagen fibers and vascular proliferation in the papillary dermis has been established. The presence of melanophages has been noted.

One of the objections that can be raised against most of these criteria mentioned in Table 1 is that they have not been well defined qualitatively, let alone quantitatively. Therefore we have further defined them, as will be discussed in section III.A.

III. THE METHODOLOGY OF EFFICACY STUDIES

Efficacy studies can only be executed properly if (1) the diagnostic criteria are well-defined and (2) the design of the study is sound, i.e., comparing well-defined patient and control populations and using a multivariat statistical analysis. We have previously reported on a study using this approach.[13] Therefore, we will confine ourselves here to a brief description.

A. THE DEFINITION OF THE HISTOPATHOLOGICAL CRITERIA

The features mentioned in Table 1 were further defined regarding both qualitative (present, absent) and semiquantitative (slight, moderate, marked) aspects. A specification of the elaborated criteria is given in Tables 2, 3, and 4. Unless specified otherwise, features have been scored in the following way: "easy to find", "to be looked for", or "absent". Nevoid lesions showing ascension of atypical melanocytes up into the granular layer were diagnosed as melanoma *in situ* and were therefore excluded from the current series.

B. THE DESIGN OF THE STUDY

The presence of a diagnostic histopathologic feature can be regarded as a diagnostic test. The efficacy of a diagnostic test is its ability to indicate the presence or absence of a disease and is statistically expressed in four indices (sensitivity, specificity, accuracy for positive prediction, and accuracy for negative prediction), each having a maximum value of 100%.[12] To establish efficacy of a test these indices should be examined in lesions from both a broad range of patients with the disease (diseased group) and in a broad range of individuals without the disease (comparative group).

TABLE 2
Further Definition of Histologic Features Used as Criteria Required for the Diagnosis of Dysplastic Nevus

Features of Architectural Atypia

Junctional activity
- Markedly increased when the number of melanocytes is equal to or larger than the number of basal keratinocytes, either as single cells or as loose aggregates, along at least three adjacent rete ridges in the lesion
- Moderate or slight when the number of melanocytes is less

Melanocytic preference for the rete ridges
- Totally absent
- Focally absent
- Present

Configuration of the junctional nests
- Irregular when the contours are undulated
- Regular when the contours are smooth

Bridging of rete ridges
- Present
- Absent

TABLE 3
Further Definition of Histologic Features Used as Criteria Required for the Diagnosis of Dysplastic Nevus

Features of Cellular Atypia

Large prominent melanocytes
- Present when the size of the melanocytes is larger than in adjacent perilesional skin
- Absent when the size is equal or smaller

Dusty melanin pigment
- Present
- Absent

Nuclear pleomorphism
- Present when melanocytic nuclei show a greater variation in size and shape than those in adjacent perilesional skin
- Absent when the variation is equal to or less

Large melanocytic nuclei
- Present when the size of melanocytic nuclei is equal to or larger than the size of the nuclei of neighboring keratinocytes
- Absent when the size is smaller

Prominent melanocytic nucleoli
- Present when at least one third the size of an erythrocyte
- Absent when the size is smaller

Prominent retraction artifact
- Present
- Absent

1. Diseased Group: Group A

From 36 patients with the familial or nonfamilial DN syndrome who visited the pigmented lesion clinic at University Hospital in Leiden, 62 DN removed for diagnostic purposes were reviewed histologically. The diagnosis DN syndrome was based on the presence of clinically and histologically evident DN. The histologic diagnosis was based on the presence of cellular and architectural features of atypia combined with a stromal reaction.

Thirty-one of these DN were removed from 18 patients with familial DN syndrome;[14] 7 of these patients had one or more melanomas in their history. From the 18 patients with nonfamilial DN syndrome, 31 lesions were removed; 6 patients had a history of melanoma.

TABLE 4
Further Definition of Histologic Features Used as Criteria Required for the Diagnosis of Dysplastic Nevus

Stromal Reactions

Lymphocytic infiltrate
  Marked when bandlike
  Moderate when aggregate-like
  Slight when only perivascular
Fibroplasia
  Present when the number of fibroblasts and/or the amount of collagen fibers is increased compared to adjacent perilesional dermis
  Absent when equal to or less
Angio(neo)genesis
  Present when the number of vascular structures is increased compared to adjacent perilesional dermis
  Absent when equal to or less
Melanophages
  Present
  Absent

Forty-six nevi were localized on the trunk and 16 on the extremities. The diameter of the lesions removed was measured.

2. Comparative Group: Group B

As a sample of the general population, 326 melanocytic nevi removed from 54 individuals were examined histologically. These lesions were derived from 658 pigmented lesions removed from 67 routine autopsy cases of Caucasians. Exclusion of all the histologically confirmed ephelides, keratoses, fibromas, or hemangiomas yielded 608 lesions. Because of the relative preponderance of dermal nevi (n = 79) and senile lentigines (n = 205) as compared to group A, we decided to exclude these lesions also. The melanocytic nevi were removed from 18 females and 36 males. Of the individuals examined 45% had died from cardiovascular disease, 36% from cancer, and 19% from other causes. In 13% of the cases there was a history of recent hormonal or cytostatic treatment.

Lesions smaller than 1 mm and lesions localized on the face, neck, upper chest, and back of the hands were not removed. The number of lesions removed from one individual ranged from 1 to 18; 42% were localized on the trunk, 50% on the extremities, and 8% elsewhere (neck and genital region). The maximal dimension of every lesion was registered.

C. HISTOPATHOLOGIC EXAMINATION

From 388 nevi (62 from group A and 326 from group B) ten 4-μm thick hematoxylin and eosin stained serial paraffin sections per lesion were examined histologically by four observers. The skin lesions removed from autopsy cases showed only mild signs of autolysis that did not interfere with histologic interpretation. The histologic type of the lesions was determined; the types were divided into junctional melanocytic nevi and compound melanocytic nevi. The histopathologic criteria (divided into architectural atypia, cellular atypia, and stromal reactions) used, are mentioned in Tables 2, 3, and 4.

D. STATISTICAL ANALYSIS

We have examined six architectural, six cellular, and four stromal features, most of which were scored semiquantitatively (see Tables 2, 3, and 4). The observed differences between the two groups were analyzed for significance using the chi-square test.

From these data, sensitivity, specificity, and predictive values could be calculated using cross tables and interpreting each diagnostic test positive when a feature was present. For a feature scored semiquantitatively two different values were given: one based on the decision *present vs. absent*, and one based on *markedly or moderately present vs. slightly present or absent*. By means of cross tables and the chi-square test we investigated a possible relation between the presence of each of the histopathologic criteria in lesions derived from every individual and sex and the use of recent hormonal or cytostatic therapy.

A linear discriminant analysis[15] was done to investigate which histologic criteria and, in what order, were capable of discriminating DN from common melanocytic nevi, and how often a correct classification could be made using these criteria.

IV. THE EFFICACY OF HISTOPATHOLOGIC CRITERIA REQUIRED FOR THE DIAGNOSIS OF DYSPLASTIC NEVUS

Statistical analysis showed that all the features mentioned differed significantly ($p < 0.001$) in frequency in groups A and B, except for the presence of melanophages in the dermis. For this reason, this feature was left out for further analysis. The sensitivity, the specificity, and the predictive values (given in percentages) of the histologic features diagnostic for DN are summarized in a previous report.[12] The results indicate that the efficacy of most diagnostic features if used singly is limited, due to either low sensitivity, low specificity, or low predictive values. If a feature was scored semiquantitatively, higher values for specificity and positive prediction could be reached when this feature was scored as positive and only when it was prominent. However, this implied a lower sensitivity and a lower negative predictive value.

In descending order, features (used dichotomously, i.e., present vs. absent) with a reasonable sensitivity (>80%) are pleomorphism of melanocytic nuclei, lymphocytic infiltrate, fibroplasia, prominent melanocytes, angioneogenesis, irregularity of nests, absence of melanocytic preference for the rete ridges, and prominent retraction artifacts. In descending order, features (used dichotomously) with reasonable specificity (>80%) are bridging, impairment of maturation, dusty melanin pigment, markedly increased junctional activity, large melanocytic nuclei, prominent nucleoli, irregularity of nests, nuclear pleomorphism, and absence of preference for the rete ridges. Only bridging and dusty melanin pigment are features with a high positive predictive value, whereas all features tested have a high negative predictive value.

The results of linear discriminant analysis showed that in descending order, the four most discriminating histopathologic features are the presence of dusty melanin pigment, irregular nests, markedly increased junctional activity, and large melanocytic nuclei. With these four features, 95% of the lesions can be assigned to the correct group. Using stepwise selection, the results indicated that the other features had hardly any additional discriminating ability. Performing the same procedure on a group of 90 nevi randomly selected from each individual (i.e., 36 from group A and 54 from group B) yielded the same findings. Using combinations of these four most discriminating criteria, high values for sensitivity, specificity, positive prediction, and negative prediction can be reached.

However, if we would include the lesions with only slight atypia and accept the presence of slight cellular or architectural atypia in combination with a mild perivascular infiltrate to be sufficient for the diagnosis of DN, we would find one or more DN in 46% of our autopsy cases. If fibroplasia and angioneogenesis are added as obligatory criteria, still 15% of our autopsy cases would have one or more DN.

The main purpose of this study was to estimate sensitivity, specificity, and predictive values of histologic features reported to be diagnostic for DN. These indices were calculated by assessing the frequencies of the histologic diagnostic features in two groups of nevocellular nevi.

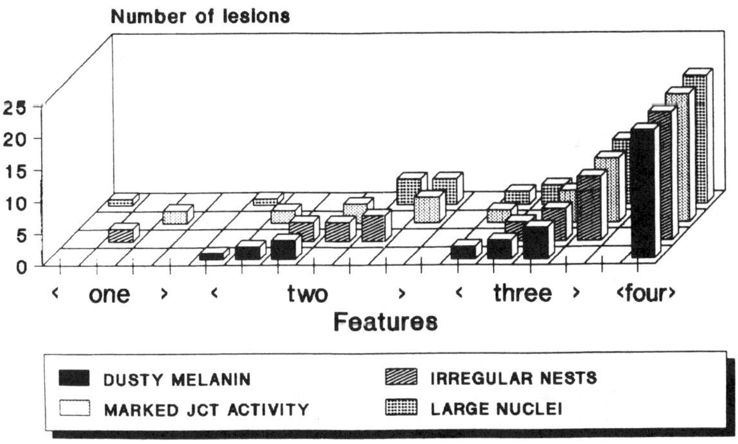

FIGURE 4. Prevalence of the four most discriminating histopathologic features in 62 dysplastic nevi studied. Numbers at the horizontal axis indicate lesions with one feature (lanes 1 to 3), two features (lanes 5 to 10), three features (lanes 12 to 15), or four features (lane 17).

A group of clinically suspect and histologically confirmed DN derived from patients with the DN syndrome[14] served as the diseased group in which diagnosis can be assumed to be certain. A series of melanocytic nevi that had been removed from consecutive autopsy cases and were not selected for features of dysplasia served as a comparative group. We are aware of the fact that, in the control group, disease cannot be excluded because we may expect an incidence of 2 to 8% of DN in the general population; this number is mainly based on clinical studies. The autopsy group was chosen for this comparative study because we consider it as a representative sample of the general population, of which the causes of death are not related to the frequency of melanocytic nevi. In addition, our study may provide information on the prevalence of histologically proven DN in the general population.

As could be expected, the efficacy of the single diagnostic feature is limited, due to low sensitivity, low specificity, or low predictive values. Discriminant analysis showed that, in decreasing order, the presence of dustlike melanin pigment, irregular nests, markedly increased junctional activity, and nuclei larger than or as large as overlying keratinocytes are the most discriminating features. All four criteria were present in 20 DN lesions, three in 23, two in 14, and one in 5 (see Figure 4). When combinations of two or more of these criteria were used, a high degree of discrimination between both groups could be reached. To avoid overestimation, the histologic diagnosis of DN should be based on a combination of strictly defined criteria.

If all major histopathologic features described as diagnostic for DN (cellular and/or architectural atypia, lymphocytic infiltrate, fibroplasia, and angioneogenesis) were used in the nevi of our autopsy group, 15% of these individuals would have one or more DN. Therefore, we emphasize that it is necessary to use a combination of criteria with the most discriminating ability. When we use combinations of two or more of the four most discriminating features mentioned in Table 3 and add lymphocytic infiltrate as an obligatory diagnostic criterion, an even higher diagnostic accuracy is reached (sensitivity 92%, specificity 98%, positive predictive value 89%, and negative predictive value 98%). These figures could be even higher if they would have been corrected for the occurrence of dysplastic nevi in the autopsy population. The prevalence of histologically proven DN in this population would be about 10% (7/67 individuals), if the combinations of criteria mentioned are accepted as diagnostic and if group B is considered as a representative sample of the general population. Our estimation of 10% is in agreement with earlier statements based on clinical examinations.[5,16-18]

TABLE 5
Proposed Histopathologic Classification of Dysplastic Nevi

Number of histopathologic criteria[a]	Classification
One	DN, slight atypia
Two or three	DN, moderate atypia
All four	DN, marked atypia
All four plus ascension into granular layer	Melanoma *in situ*

[a] Most discriminating criteria described (see text).

Conceivably, DN with marked architectural and/or cellular atypia are the most likely to progress to *in situ* or invasive melanoma. Therefore, recognition of these DN is important. In our opinion, markedly atypical DN should have at least the four features with the most discriminating ability, i.e., *markedly increased junctional activity, irregular nests, large melanocytic nuclei,* and *dustlike melanin.* Such nevi with marked atypia were common (in 18 of 36 patients) in the diseased group (A), but were not found in all 54 individuals of the comparative group (B). Therefore, the presence of a DN with marked atypia should be considered as an indication of an increased risk of getting melanoma.

V. OBSERVER STUDIES ON THE USE OF THE HISTOPATHOLOGIC CRITERIA SELECTED

In order to further assess the efficacy of the histopathologic diagnostic approach based on the criteria selected, we have set up an inter- and intra-observer study. For this purpose a series of 20 common nevocellular nevi, 60 dysplastic nevi with different degree of atypia, and 20 Clark level I (melanoma *in situ*) or level II superficial spreading melanomas were selected. The study aims at establishing not only the reproducibility of diagnosing dysplastic nevi, but also of grading these lesions. The proposed grading system is based on the four most discriminating histopathologic criteria mentioned in Section IV (see Table 5). If next to these criteria of DN, ascension of atypical melanocytes into the granular layer of the epidermis is found, the lesion is classified as melanoma *in situ* that has arisen in a DN.

During a pilot study preceding the observer study, we noted that the histopathologic criteria selected were less suitable in acrolentiginous lesions and in nevocellular nevi of prepubertal children. Based on the experience of some experts,[19] the diagnosis DN in acrolentiginous lesions should be restricted to those having cellular atypia. Architectural atypia per se in such lesions, even including ascension of melanocytes up to the granular layer does not warrant this diagnosis. The same holds true for nevocellular nevi of prepubertal children. It remains to be defined from what age DN can be diagnosed. These exceptions to the application of the histopathologic criteria reemphasize the point that the diagnosis DN can only be made in a proper clinicopathologic context.[20,21]

VI. CONCLUSIONS

Based on the foregoing discussions we conclude that:

1. The dysplastic nevus has distinctive histopathologic features.
2. In a proper clinicopathologic context a histopathologic diagnosis of dysplastic nevus can be made only by using a combination of well-defined criteria.
3. The estimated prevalence of histologically proven dysplastic nevi in the general population is 10%.

4. Further inter- and intra-observer studies are needed in order to reach consensus on the histologic criteria and to assess the reproducibility of the histopathologic diagnosis. This is not only relevant for the clinical situation, but also for future epidemiological surveys.

ACKNOWLEDGMENTS

The authors would like to thank Mr. T. van Eupen for preparing the microphotographs and Ms. Y. Stammes for typing the manuscript.

REFERENCES

1. **Elder, D. E., Goldman, S. C., et al.,** Dysplastic nevus syndromes: a phenotypic association of sporadic cutaneous melanoma, *Cancer,* 1787, 1980.
2. **Elder, D. E., Greene, M. H., Bondi, E. E., et al.,** Acquired melanocytic nevi and melanoma: the dysplastic nevus syndrome, in *Pathology of Malignant Melanoma,* Ackerman, A. B., Ed., Masson, New York, 1981.
3. **Reed, R. J., Clark, W. H., Jr., and Mihm, M. C., Jr.,** Premalignant melanocytic dysplasia, in *Pathology of Malignant Melanoma,* Ackerman, A. B., Ed., Masson, New York, 1981.
4. **Cochran, A. J.,** Histology of "borderline" and atypical cutaneous malignant melanoma, *Pigment Cell,* Vol. 6, S. Karger, Basel, 1983.
5. Precursors to malignant melanoma, Consensus Development Conference, National Institutes of Health, Bethesda, *JAMA,* 251, 1864, 1983.
6. **Sagebiel, R. W.,** Diagnosis and management of premalignant melanocytic proliferations, *Pathology,* 17, 285, 1985.
7. **Rubin, E. and Farber, J. L.,** Cell Injury, in *Pathology,* Rubin, E. and Farber, J. L., Eds., Lippincott, Philadelphia, 1988, 2.
8. **Rywlin, M.,** Dysplasia. On the terminology of atypical intraepithelial proliferations, *Am. J. Dermatopathol.,* 3, 183, 1981.
9. **Ackerman, A. B. and Mihara, J.,** Dysplasia, dysplastic melanocytes, dysplastic nevi, the dysplastic nevus syndrome, and the relation between dysplastic nevi and malignant melanomas, *Hum. Pathol.,* 16, 87, 1985.
10. **Rahbari, H. and Mehregan, A. M.,** Sporadic atypical mole syndrome. A report of five non-familial B-K syndrome like cases and histopathologic findings, *Arch. Dermatol.,* 117, 329, 1981.
11. **Ruiter, D. J., Bergman, W., Steijlen, P. M., et al.,** Histopathological aspects of dysplastic nevi, in *Cutaneous Melanoma and Precursor Lesions,* Ruiter, D. J., Welvaart, K., and Ferrone, S., Eds., Martinius Nijhoff, Boston, 1984.
12. **Steijlen, P. M., Bergman, W., Hermans, J., Scheffer, E., van Vloten, W. A., and Ruiter, D. J.,** The efficacy of histopathological criteria required for diagnosing dysplastic naevi, *Histopathology,* 12, 289, 1988.
13. **Ransohoff, D. F. and Feinstein, A. R.,** Problems of spectrum and bias in evaluating the efficacy of diagnostic tests, *N. Engl. J. Med.,* 299, 926, 1978.
14. **Bergman, W., Palan, A., and Went, L. N.,** Clinical and genetic studies in six Dutch kindreds with the dysplastic naevus syndrome, *Ann. Hum. Genet.,* 50, 249, 1986.
15. **Hull, C. H.,** *SPSS-X Users Guide,* McGraw-Hill, New York, 1983.
16. **Crutcher, W. A. and Sagebiel, R. W.,** Prevalence of dysplastic naevi in a community practice, *Lancet,* i.i., 729, 1984.
17. **Nordlund, J. J., Kirkwood, J., and Forget, B. M.,** Demographic study of clinically atypical (dysplastic) nevi in patients with melanoma and comparison subjects, *Cancer Res.,* 45, 1855, 1985.
18. **MacKie, R. M., English, J., Aitchinson, T. C., et al.,** The number and distribution of benign pigmented moles (melanocytic naevi) in a healthy population, *Br. J. Dermatol.,* 113, 167, 1985.
19. **Mihm, M. C., Jr.,** *Personal communication,* 1987.
20. **Clark, W. H., Jr.,** The dysplastic nevus syndrome editorial, *Arch. Dermatol.,* 124, 1207, 1988.
21. **Elder, D. E.,** Dysplastic nevus syndrome—biological significance, *Semin. Oncol.,* 15, 529, 1988.

Chapter 6

HLA AND MALIGNANT MELANOMA

Florence M. Demenais

TABLE OF CONTENTS

I. INTRODUCTION

The identification of a precursor to cutaneous malignant melanoma (CMM)[1-3] has provided new opportunities to seek for genetic marker(s) closely linked to melanoma susceptibility gene(s), which can lead to detection of high-risk persons. The precursor lesions, or dysplastic nevi (DN), have been found in CMM patients belonging to multiplex families and their relatives. The vertical familial transmission of this syndrome, known as B-K mole or familial atypical multiple mole melanoma (FAMMM) syndrome, has suggested a dominant pattern of inheritance. Besides other possible genomic locations of a melanoma susceptibility gene,[4] a prominent candidate is the region of the human major histocompatibility complex (HLA), located on the short arm of chromosome 6. As well known, the HLA region is composed of several genes which play a role in the immune function, and a few immunologic abnormalities have been reported in members of high-risk melanoma families.[5-7] Furthermore, patients with acquired or inherited immunodeficiencies are at increasing risk of developing melanoma.[8-9] The tumors themselves express not only specific antigens but also HLA-A, -B, -C, and -DR determinants that could influence the immune processes.[10-11]

After outlining the main characteristics of the HLA system and the statistical methods used to detect the involvement of HLA in a disease, a possible role of HLA in malignant melanoma will be discussed.

II. THE HLA SYSTEM

A. GENETIC CHARACTERISTICS

The HLA region is made up of several closely linked loci located on the short arm of chromosome 6. These loci are designated HLA-A, -B, -C, -DR, -DP, and -DQ. In addition, complement factors C2, C4 (C4A and C4B), and Bf (factor B of properdin) are also located within this complex (see Figure 1). Each of the A, B, and C loci code for polymorphic polypeptide chain, which is combined with the unvariant β-2 microglobulin controlled by a gene on chromosome 15, to form HLA Class I molecules. The DR, DP, and DQ loci code for two different polypeptide chains, alpha and beta, to constitute Class II factors. The recent progress in molecular biology has allowed a detailed mapping of this region.[12] The factors involved in the complement cascade are called HLA Class III factors. Besides the Class I, II, and III factors, the HLA system contains the genes for 21-hydroxylase, the tumor necrosis factor (TNFA) and lymphotoxin (TNFB), and a gene causing idiopathic hemochromatosis. Each person has two alleles at each HLA locus coding for two antigens which are expressed independently (codominant). All the HLA loci are tightly linked, the recombination between adjacent loci is less than 1%. The entire set of HLA-A, -B, -C, and -D genes located on one chromosome is called a haplotype, which is usually inherited by children as a unit. One important characteristic of the HLA genes is their high degree of polymorphism (i.e., several alleles exist at each locus in the population), which makes HLA an ideal marker for genetic studies. Indeed, two parents, taken at random from the population, are likely to be both heterozygous and different, and thus informative in family studies. The frequencies of HLA antigens vary also among ethnic groups.[13-14] Another important feature of the HLA region is the pronounced linkage disequilibrium between the alleles at nearby loci. The joint frequency of two alleles at two different loci is significantly different from the value expected in a random mating population at equilibrium, i.e., the product of the individual allelic frequencies. This causes the observed associations among the HLA antigens themselves.

B. TYPING METHODS

Determination of HLA-A, -B, and -C antigens is performed by the microlymphocytotoxicity test on peripheral lymphocytes.[15] The HLA-DR antigens are typed, using the same

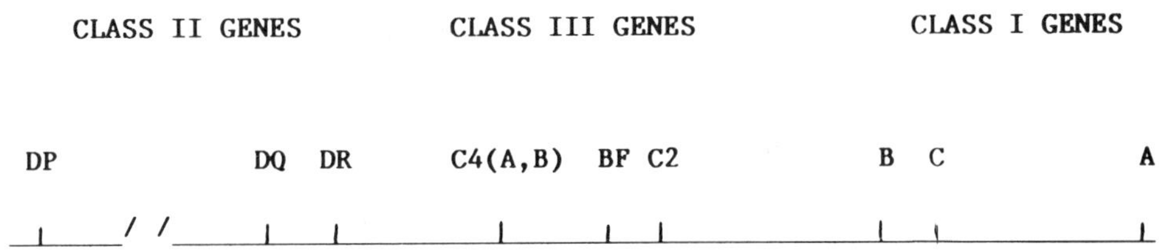

FIGURE 1. Map of the HLA region on the short arm of chromosome 6.

test on B lymphocytes. B cells are initially isolated by the rosetting of sheep cells[16] or the nylon wool adherence.[17] Standardization of the HLA testing and adoption of a nomenclature of HLA antigens have been the results from several international workshops, started since 1964. HLA-A and -B antigens were first identified,[18] whereas HLA-C and -DR loci were only introduced in 1975, at the Sixth International Histocompatibility Workshop.[19] It should therefore be kept in mind that, in comparing the reports of HLA and disease associations, the definition of HLA antigens has gradually evolved over time. A current nomenclature of HLA antigens can be found in the report of the Ninth Histocompatibility Workshop.[14]

C. BIOLOGICAL FUNCTION

Class I and II factors are involved in the thymus-dependent immune response at the cellular cooperation level. Briefly, the protein antigens are first processed by the antigen-presenting cells (mainly monocytes and macrophages), and then bound in the groove on Class II molecules to be transported to the cell surface and presented to the T-cell receptor (Ti) on T-helper (Th) lymphocytes. Th lymphocytes with Ti receptor specific for the peptide-Class II combination become activated and help B lymphocytes to differentiate into plasma cells producing antibodies toward the original antigen, leading to inactivation of the invading microorganism. Th lymphocytes can also induce precursors of cytotoxic/suppressive T (Tc/s) lymphocytes to become actively cytotoxic (Tc) or suppressive (Ts). Tc lymphocytes can kill virus-infected cells. Ts lymphocytes can suppress the immune response and prevent it from bolting. Various hormones, called lymphokines, are involved during this activation process. These cellular interactions are HLA restricted: Class II molecules are required for the macrophage-Th lymphocytes interactions, whereas Class I molecules are necessary for the virus-infected cells-Tc lymphocytes interactions. The ability of HLA molecules to bind a given antigen peptide will result in a more or less strong immune response. Class III factors have also been shown to play a role in the immune lysis.[20]

III. HLA AND DISEASE: STATISTICAL METHODOLOGY

A. POPULATION DATA ANALYSIS

HLA and disease associations are primarily detected by comparing the frequencies of HLA antigens in a group of patients and suitable controls, i.e., unrelated healthy individuals matched for sex, age, race, and other appropriate variables. For each HLA antigen tested, the frequency of this antigen is compared between patients and controls, using a 2×2 contingency table and the usual chi-squared test with one degree of freedom (df). An alternative method, originally proposed by Woolf[21] and then modified by Haldane,[22] tests if the relative risk departs significantly from unity. Let h and k be the number of patients respectively positive and negative for a given antigen; let H and K be the number of controls respectively positive and negative for this antigen. The relative risk (or more exactly the odd ratio) is $x = hK/Hk$. Its significance is tested by $X^2 = y^2/V(y)$ with 1 df, where $y = \ln(x)$ and $V(y) = 1/h + 1/k + 1/H + 1/K$. The type I error or p value associated with the chi-squared test is 0.05, which means that in 5% of comparisons the relative risk significantly deviates from unity by chance. A problem in testing HLA-disease associations is that the same data are used to compare all the typed antigens, and that few tests can be significant only by chance. One way to circumvent the problem of multiple testing is to multiply the *p* value corresponding to the calculated chi-squared for each antigen comparison by the total number of antigens compared.[23] If any corrected *p* value is still less than 5%, then the antigen is considered significantly associated with the disease. However, such correction is very conservative, and another way to confirm an association is to repeat the studies on the same disease and to test particularly for the antigen reported associated by the first study without any correction. General methods have been recently developed to make multiple testing on several HLA antigens simultaneously.[24-25] After eliminating a possible bias due to the stratification of the population studied (e.g., patients belong to a group of individuals in which an antigen is more frequent by chance), HLA-disease associations can be caused by the following mechanisms:

1. The HLA locus is directly involved in the susceptibility to the disease (pleiotropy); it can act alone or in interaction with another gene on another chromosome to cause the disease (epistasis).
2. The HLA locus is in linkage disequilibrium with another tightly linked susceptibility locus (disease locus or immune response gene).

Therefore, to confirm the genetic cause of an HLA-disease association, family studies are required.

B. FAMILY DATA ANALYSIS

Two types of methods are used to search for a genetic involvement of the HLA system in a disease: a method based on sib pairs or sibship data and the classical linkage analysis based on the lod score method applied to the whole family data.

1. Sib-Pair Method

This method has been used for most HLA-associated diseases, which are not inherited in a simple Mendelian fashion, since it does not require the specification of a particular mode of inheritance for the disease. The sib-pair test was originally proposed by Penrose,[26] and since then, many variations have been developed[27-28] for a review. It will be only briefly outlined, since it has not been applied to the melanoma data. The sib-pair method tests whether the observed distribution of parental HLA haplotypes among affected sib pairs differs significantly from the distribution expected under the null hypothesis of independent segregation between the disease locus and the HLA region. A significant difference indicates the genetic involvement of the HLA system in the disease.

2. Lod Score Method

This method studies the cosegregation of a disease and a marker in the families as a whole. It provides not only a test for the presence of linkage, but also an estimate of the recombination fraction (i.e., genetic distance) between the disease gene and the marker (HLA) locus. The distance between two genes on the same chromosome is assumed to be related to the number of crossing overs that occur between them during meiosis. Since a crossing over corresponds genetically to a recombination, an increased distance between two loci is expected to be associated with a higher recombination fraction, Θ. A Θ value of 0.50 corresponds to the independence between the two loci (i.e., the two loci are on two different chromosomes or on the same chromosome but far enough apart so that their segregation is independent). Linkage analysis is based on the lod score method, originally described by Morton[29] and then generalized.[30] The lod score method measures the odds of linkage for different recombination values ($\Theta = 0.0, 0.05, \ldots 0.45$) vs. no linkage ($\Theta = 0.50$). A lod score of 3.0 (odds of 1000 to 1) is considered as significant evidence in favor of linkage, and a lod score of -2.0 is taken as evidence against linkage at a given Θ value. A lod score of 2.0 is already considered as suggestive of linkage. The recombination fraction at which the lod score is maximum is the maximum likelihood estimate of the recombination fraction between the disease susceptibility gene and the HLA gene. Lod scores on several families and from different studies can be sequentially added until a definite statement with respect to presence (total lod score >3.0) or absence (total lod score <-2.0) of linkage can be made. A test of homogeneity among families or studies can be performed by substracting the maximum lod score on the pooled data and the sum of the individual maximum lod scores obtained for each family or for a subgroup of families.[31] Other tests of homogeneity have been also proposed.[30]

One disadvantage of this linkage method is that the mode of inheritance of the disease is assumed to be known, following a simple Mendelian transmission. Several theoretical studies have been conducted to explore the consequences of a false assumption. All of them have shown that the linkage test itself is robust against a misspecification of the mode of inheritance (there is no false conclusion of linkage); however, the estimate of the recombination fraction can be strongly biased.[32] Several computer programs have been developed to allow calculation of lod scores in pedigrees for various modes of inheritance. The computer program LIPED[33-34] was used for all melanoma data.

IV. HLA AND MALIGNANT MELANOMA

A. POPULATION DATA ANALYSIS

The search for association between CMM and HLA Class I antigens (A or B) has led to numerous population studies, especially of Caucasian North Americans and Europeans (Belgians, English, French, Norwegians, Danes, and Italians).[13] No consistent association was found in the combined data. A reduced frequency of HLA-B5 was first reported by Clark et al.,[35] which was apparently caused by a specific masking factor. The largest number of patients studied (n = 226) did not lead to any significant association with HLA-A and -B antigens.[36] However, in a series of 140 melanoma patients from Italy, Pellegris et al.[37] found a significant increase of HLA-B40 (15% in patients vs. 4.09% in 904 controls; $p = 5.6 \times 10^{-7}$) and a significant decrease of HLA-Bw35 (12.85% in patients vs. 28.13% in 853 controls; $p = 1.6 \times 10^{-4}$). The increase of HLA-B40 was reported again once in 145 patients from Metropolitan New York (14.5% vs. 8.8% in 388 controls), particularly in those with poor prognosis of the disease.[38] No particular association was found when the patients were subdivided into subgroups according to sex, survival at 5 years,[39] or presence or not of clinical evidence of melanoma.[37] However, a significant increase of HLA-A9 was observed in severe forms of the cancer, especially in the metastatic or relapsing forms.[40]

D locus typing was first performed on 44 Norwegian patients,[41] and no significant association was found. A similar negative result was reported by Nathanson et al.[42-43] in 236 American Caucasian patients or in subgroups based on sex and stage of cancer. However, Barger et al.[44] identified a significant association of CMM with DR4, particularly in a low-risk subgroup, based on their clinically defined risk status at diagnosis. A significantly positive association with DR5 was found in a group of patients with poor prognosis from the New York series[38] (35% in 21 patients vs. 20.5% in 176 controls) and in a subgroup of German patients presenting the superficial spreading melanoma (SSM) histologic type (46.3% in 67 patients vs. 26.9% in 847 controls; $p = 0.0019$ and corrected $p < 0.05$).[45] DR5 was also reported to be associated with other malignancies.[38]

B. FAMILY STUDIES

The cosegregation of CMM and HLA in families was only studied by linkage analyses, which require, as mentioned earlier, the specification of a monogenic mode of inheritance for the disease.

1. Mode of Inheritance of CMM and/or DN

Over the years, familial aggregation of CMM has been attributed either to polygenic inheritance[46-47] or to a dominant single gene with reduced penetrance.[48-49] The recognition of the FAMMM syndrome, showing vertical transmission, favored the dominant pattern of inheritance in these high-risk families.[50-51] However, sporadic cases of precursor lesions, with or without melanoma, have also been described.[52-53] Their frequency is high, since Crutcher and Sagebiel[54] reported that 4.8% of 881 consecutive patients followed for dermatologic problems unrelated to pigmented skin lesions had histologically proven dysplastic nevi. In addition, a possible polygenic inheritance of DN was discussed by Happle et al.[55] A formal genetic analysis was conducted in 14 Caucasian American pedigrees with at least two melanoma cases and displaying the FAMM syndrome in all of them.[4] The maximum likelihood method of segregation analysis, using the transmission probability model of Elston and Stewart,[56] was applied to these data to test the hypothesis of single gene transmission of the disease. Whereas the familial distribution of CMM itself was consistent with an autosomal dominant mode of inheritance, Mendelian segregation at one locus for the phenotype defined by CMM or DN or both did not fit the data. The probability for a heterozygote to transmit the deleterious allele was estimated at 1.0, greater than the expected value of 0.5, under the Mendelian transmission hypothesis. This could be attributed to the presence of phenocopies (nonfamilial DN), an ascertainment bias and/or a more complex genetic mechanism. However, this analysis assumed the same penetrance (probability for gene carriers to manifest the disease) for both DN and CMM traits and did not allow tests of alternative genetic models (two locus or polygenic models). When the data were reanalyzed,[57] using a life table analysis,[58] the lifetime incidence of melanoma in the sibs and offspring of DN-affected individuals was estimated to be 46%, consistent with a highly penetrant dominant gene. Conversely, the probability of showing DN in first degree relatives of CMM patients was estimated to be 54%, not statistically different from 50%. Linkage analysis, carried out between the two traits DN and CMM, assumed to be each determined by a fully penetrant dominant gene, led to a significant positive lod score (3.857) at a recombination rate Θ of 8%. Θ did not differ significantly from zero, suggesting a unique pleiotropic gene for the two traits. However, the estimated Θ value of 8% could be also due to a more complex genetic mechanism, such that genetic heterogeneity or a two-locus model for the cancer itself. The gene causing familial DN may be one among other genetic determinants of CMM. Indeed, families with familial CMM are known, which do not show the DN syndrome.[59] Recently, the genetic study of six Dutch kindreds with the dysplastic naevus syndrome has suggested that the penetrance of the DNS gene may not be as high and varying among families.[60]

2. Linkage Analyses

Since the relationship and mode of inheritance of CMM and DN are not as clearly defined, linkage analyses have considered the different following patterns for the disease phenotype studied:

1. Only individuals with DN (with or without CMM) are affected.
2. All individuals displaying any of the clinical form (DN or CMM or both) are affected.
3. Only individuals showing CMM are affected.

TABLE 1
Data Submitted to Linkage Analysis

Origin of the data	Reference	Trait studied DN	DN/CMM	CMM	Total no. of families
Australia	61	–	–	+	1
France	63	+	+	+	7
WKS9[a]	62	+	+	+	22
U.S. (NIH)	64	–	+	+	11
Pub. data set[b]	64	–	–	+	19

Note: DN = dysplastic nevi, CMM = cutaneous malignant melanoma.

[a] WKS9 identifies data analyzed for the Ninth Histocompatibility Workshop.
[b] Pub. data set identifies a set of published data reanalyzed by the NIH group (as explained in the text).

TABLE 2
Linkage Analyses Between HLA and a Dominant Gene for Dysplastic Nevi (DN)

Origin of the data	Trait parameter values Gene Frequency	Penetrance	Conclusions
France	0.001	0.50	Linkage excluded (Θ ≤5%)
WKS9[a]	0.001	0.50	Linkage excluded (Θ ≤10%)

[a] WKS9 identifies data analyzed for the Ninth Histocompatibility Workshop.

Table 1 summarizes which traits (1), (2), and/or (3) have been analyzed by each study, as well as the respective sample size. The first linkage analysis concerned an Australian kindred,[61] which did not report the presence of DN among family members. However, the kindred in question was included in the workshop series (WKS9)[62] that we analyzed and displayed the FAMMM syndome. All the pedigrees from the French[63] and American (NIH)[64] series had the FAMMM syndrome. The 11 NIH families were part of the data submitted to segregation analysis.[4] The 22 families pooled for the Ninth Histocompatibility Workshop (WKS9)[62] were from different parts of the world: they included 10 families with the DN phenotype and 17 families had family members with multinaevomatosis. The so-called published data set (reanalyzed by the NIH group),[64] included the Australian pedigree, the seven French pedigrees, and in addition six Italian[65] and five German families[45] reported to have affected sib-pairs sharing at least one HLA haplotype, but without lod score computation. Linkage analyses were all conducted, assuming a dominant pattern of inheritance for each of the traits studied. The parameters (gene frequency and penetrance) at the disease locus varied according to the studies. As mentioned above, misspecification of the mode of inheritance, including wrong parameter values, may bias the recombination fraction but does not lead to a spurious inference of linkage.

The results of linkage analyses between HLA and trait (1) are presented in Table 2. Only, those trait parameter values which led to the most significant results and were also comparable with those of other studies, are shown in Table 2, although the lod scores were computed for varying gene frequency (0.0001 to 0.30) and penetrance values (0.05 to 0.90). Close linkage between HLA and DN could be excluded, at a distance less than or equal to five cross-over (c.o.) units (French series) or even ten c.o. units (WKS9 series), assuming a low-gene frequency. When trait (2), defined by DN or CMM or both, was analyzed,

TABLE 3
Linkage Analyses Between HLA and a Dominant Gene for Dysplastic Nevi (DN) or Cutaneous Malignant Melanoma (CMM) or Both

Origin of the data	Trait parameter values		Conclusions
	Gene frequency	Penetrance	
France	0.001	0.50	Linkage excluded (Θ ≤10%)
WKS9[a]	0.001	0.50	Linkage excluded (Θ ≤10%)
U.S. (NIH)	0.003	0.99	Linkage excluded (Θ ≤30%)

[a] WKS9 identifies data analyzed for the Ninth Histocompatibility Workshop.

TABLE 4
Linkage Analyses Between HLA and a Dominant Gene for Cutaneous Malignant Melanoma (CMM)

Origin of data	Trait parameter values		Conclusions
	Gene frequency	Penetrance	
Australia	0.001	0.50	MLS : 1.25 (Θ = 10%)
France	0.001	0.05	MLS : 1.64 (Θ = 5%)
		0.50	MLS : 1.32 (Θ = 9%)
WKS9[a]	0.001	0.05	MLS : 0.94 (Θ = 21%)
		0.50	MLS : 0.71 (Θ = 23%)
U.S. (NIH)	0.003	0.99	Linkage excluded (Θ ≤30%)
Pub. data set[b]	0.003	0.99	MLS : 1.46 (Θ = 20%)

Note: MLS = maximum lod score.

[a] WKS9 identifies data analyzed for the Ninth Histocompatibility Workshop.
[b] Pub. data set identifies a set of published data reanalyzed by the NIH group (as explained in the text).

exclusion of linkage with HLA was even stronger and consistent overall data sets (see Table 3): at a distance less than or equal to 10 c.o. units in the French or WKS9 series and 30 c.o. units in the NIH series. There was no heterogeneity within each data set or between the French and WKS9 data[66] or NIH and French data,[64] respectively. When the malignant state was analyzed separately (trait [3]), the different studies yielded to discordant results (see Table 4). Again, only the parameter values leading to the most significant conclusions are presented here. Whereas, the Australian and French studies indicated a trend in favor of a possible linkage (maximum lod scores of 1.25 at Θ = 10% and 1.64 at Θ = 5%, respectively), this was not supported by the WKS9 series (maximum lod score of 0.94 at Θ = 21%). Linkage homogeneity tested within and between the French and WKS9 (including the Australian pedigree) data sets did not show any significant difference, even when all families displaying DN were compared to those without DN. Lod scores computed on the pooled data led to a maximum value of 1.78 at Θ = 20%, which is still lower than the significant level of 3.0 to establish linkage.[66] However, none of these data sets led to exclusion of linkage, whatever the trait parameters considered, except for low-gene frequency and only at Θ = 0% in the WKS9 series. Very different results were observed in the NIH data. Assuming a gene frequency of 0.003 and a very high penetrance for gene carriers of 99% with a 1% sporadic rate, linkage between a CMM gene and HLA was excluded at a value of the recombination fraction ≤30%. When the NIH pedigrees were pooled to the so-called published data set, linkage was excluded for all values of Θ ≤40%. No heterogeneity was detected within each of these data sets, but there was significant heterogeneity between the NIH families and the published group ($X^2 = 6.74$, df = 1, $p < 0.01$). A maximum lod score of 1.46 at Θ close to 20% was obtained in the published group. Different mechanisms can cause this heterogeneity in the HLA-CMM linkage. There may be more than one genetic mechanism causing familial CMM. Moreover, it may not be appropriate to use the same parameters for the disease in different data sets, since risk factors, such as skin phenotype and degree of exposure to sun, may act differently in different populations on genetically susceptible individuals. We do not think that the most likely explanation of the difference between the studies is the overreporting of positive results in the published data group, as pointed out by Bale et al.[64] The WKS9 series, gathered from various sources without any *a priori* knowledge of the results, did not lead to exclusion of linkage between CMM and HLA as did the NIH data.

V. CONCLUSIONS

In conclusion, the population data have revealed weak associations between HLA and malignant melanoma, except for severe forms of the disease. This is consistent with the findings obtained in other malignancies, where the role of HLA appears modest in comparison to the mice models.[67] The different family studies lead us to propose two hypotheses: (1) there is only one gene determining the DN phenotype or CMM or both which is not linked to the HLA system, and (2) there is a more complex mechanism involving several factors, genetic and environmental, interacting with the gene determining precursor lesions to cause the neoplastic transformation. In the latter case, the precursor lesion gene is not linked to HLA, but the HLA system might influence the progress to malignancy, probably at a late stage of tumor development. Furthermore, there may not be a ubiquitous explanation, and different mechanisms may be involved in different populations.

Linkage with other markers has been investigated and revealed a lod score of 1.56 for the rhesus blood group locus at $\Theta = 30\%$, when considering the DN/CMM phenotype but not the cancer alone.[4] Studies using restriction fragment length polymorphisms are now underway, in order to map the gene for precursor lesions. This will allow the detection of high-risk individuals in families and a better understanding of the mechanisms involved at the molecular level.

Concurrent genetic epidemiology studies in a large sample of families — selected systematically through CMM patients, and considered not only for the affected status but also for the major environmental risk factors in family members — may provide some insight into the genetic mechanisms causing this cancer.

REFERENCES

1. **Clark, W. H., Jr., Reimer, R. R., Greene, M. H., Ainsworth, A. M., and Mastrangelo, M. J.,** Origin of familial melanoma from heritable melanocytic lesions: the B-K mole syndrome, *Arch. Dermatol.*, 114, 732, 1978.
2. **Lynch, H. T., Frichot, B. C., and Lynch, J. F.,** Familial atypical multiple mole-melanoma syndrome, *J. Med. Genet.*, 15, 352, 1978.
3. **Reimer, R. R., Clark, W. H., Jr., Greene, M. H., Ainsworth, A., and Fraumeni, J. F., Jr.,** Precursor lesions in familial melanoma. A new genetic preneoplastic syndrome, *JAMA*, 239, 744, 1978.
4. **Greene, M. H., Goldin, L. R., Clark, Jr., W. H., Lourien, E., Kraemer, K. H., Tucker, M. A., Elder, D. E., Fraser, M. C., and Rowe, S.,** Familial cutaneous malignant melanoma: autosomal dominant trait possibly linked to the Rh locus, *Proc. Natl. Acad. Sci. U.S.A.*, 80, 6071, 1983.

5. **Dean, J., Greene, M. H., Reimer, R. R., LeSane, F. V., McKeen, E. A., Mulvihill, J. J., Blattner, W. A., Herberman, R. B., and Fraumeni, J. F., Jr.**, Immunologic abnormalities in melanoma-prone families, *JNCI*, 63, 1139, 1979.
6. **Vandenbark, A., Greene, M. H., Burger, D., Vetto, M., and Reimer, R. R.**, Immune response to melanoma extracts in three melanoma prone families, *JNCI*, 63, 1147, 1979.
7. **Hersey, P., Edwards, A., Honeyman, M., and McCarthy, W. H.**, Low natural killer cell activity in familial melanoma patients and their relatives, *Br. J. Cancer.*, 40, 113, 1981.
8. **Greene, M. H., Young, T. I., and Clark, W. H., Jr.**, Malignant melanoma in renal transplant recipients, *Lancet*, 1, 1196, 1981.
9. **Tucker, M. A., Misfeldt, D., Coleman, C. N., Clark, W. H., Jr., Rosenberg, S. A., and Kaplan, H. S.**, Cutaneous malignant melanoma following Hodgkin's disease, *Ann. Intern. Med.*, 102, 37, 1985.
10. **Ruiter, D. J., Bhan, A. K., Harrist, T. J., Sober, A. S., and Mihm, M. C.**, Major histocompatibility antigens and mononuclear inflammatory infiltrate in benign nevomelanocytic proliferations and malignant melanoma, *J. Immunol.*, 129, 2808, 1982.
11. **Brocker, E. B., Suter, L., and Sorg, C.**, HLA-DR antigen expression in primary melanomas of the skin, *J. Invest. Dermatol.*, 82, 244, 1984.
12. **Dupont, B.**, *Immunobiology of HLA*, Springer-Verlag, New York, 1989, in press.
13. **Tiwari, J. L. and Terasaki, P. I.**, *HLA and Disease Associations*, Springer-Verlag, Berlin, 1985, chap. 2.
14. **Albert, E. D., Baur, M. P., and Mayr, W. R.**, *Histocompatibility Testing 1984*, Springer-Verlag, Heidelberg, 1984.
15. **Mittal, K. K., Mickey, M. R., Singal, D. P., and Terasaki, P. I.**, Refinement of microdroplet lymphocyte cytotoxicity test, *Transplantation*, 6, 923, 1968.
16. **Van Rood, J. J., van Leeuwen, A., Keuning, J. J., and Blusse van Oud Albas, A.**, The serological recognition of the human MHC determinants using a modified cytotoxicity technique, *Tissue Antigens*, 5, 73, 1975.
17. **Danilovs, J., Ayoub, G., and Terasaki, P. I.**, B lymphocyte isolation by thrombin-nylon wool, in *Histocompatibility Testing*, 1980, Terasaki, P. I., Ed., UCLA Tissue Typing Laboratory, Los Angeles, 1980, 287.
18. **Dausset, J.**, Iso-leuco anticorps, *Acta. Haematol.*, 20, 156, 1958.
19. **Kissmeyer-Nielsen, F.**, *Histocompatibility Testing*, Munksgaard, Copenhagen, 1975.
20. **Svejgaard, A. and Ryder, L. P.**, HLA and insulin-dependent diabetes: an overview, *Genet. Epidemiol.*, 6, 1, 1989.
21. **Woolf, B.**, On estimating the relation between blood group and disease, *Ann. Hum. Genet.*, 19, 251, 1955.
22. **Haldane, J. B. S.**, The estimation and significance of the logarithm of a ratio of frequencies, *Ann. Hum. Genet.*, 20, 309, 1956.
23. **Svejgaard, A., Jersild, C., Nielsen, L. S., and Bodmer, W. F.**, HL-A antigens and disease, *Tissue Antigens*, 4, 95, 1974.
24. **Smouse, P. E. and Williams, R. C.**, Multivariate analysis of HLA-disease associations, *Biometrics*, 38, 757, 1982.
25. **Fukuda, K., Sugawa, K., Wakisaka, A., Moriuchi, J., Matsuura, N., and Sato, Y.**, Statistical detection of HLA and disease association, *Tissue Antigens*, 26, 81, 1985.
26. **Penrose, L. S.**, The detection of autosomal linkage in data which consists of pairs of brothers and sisters of unspecified parentage, *Ann. Eugen.*, 6, 133, 1935.
27. **Suarez, B. K. and Van Eerdewegh, P.**, A comparison of three affected sib-pair scoring methods to detect HLA-linked disease susceptibility genes, *Am. J. Med. Genet.*, 18, 135, 1984.
28. **Blackwelder, W. C. and Elston, R. C.**, A comparison of sib-pair linkage tests for disease susceptibility loci, *Genet. Epidemiol.*, 2, 85, 1985.
29. **Morton, N. E.**, Sequential tests for the detection of linkage, *Am. J. Hum. Genet.*, 7, 277, 1955.
30. **Ott, J.**, *Analysis of Human Genetic Linkage*, The Johns Hopkins University Press, Baltimore, 1985.
31. **Morton, N. E.**, The detection and estimation of linkage between the genes for elliptocytosis and the Rh type, *Am. J. Hum. Genet.*, 8, 80, 1956.
32. **Rice, J. and Risch, N.**, Genetic analysis of the affective disorders: summary of GAW5, *Genet. Epidemiol.*, 6, 161, 1989.
33. **Ott, J.**, Estimation of the recombination fraction in human pedigrees: efficient computation of the likelihood for human linkage studies, *Am. J. Hum. Genet.*, 26, 588, 1974.
34. **Ott, J.**, A simple scheme for the analysis of HLA linkages in pedigrees, *Ann. Hum. Genet.*, 45, 255, 1978.
35. **Clark, D. A., Necheles, T. F., Nathanson, L., Whitten, D., Silverman, E., and Flowers, A.**, Apparent HLA-A5 deficiency in human malignant melanoma: the HLA-A5 masking activity in sera of patients with progressing disease, *Isr. J. Med. Sci.*, 10, 836, 1974.

36. **Terasaki, P. I., Perdue, S. T., and Mickey, M. R.,** HLA frequencies in cancer: a second study, in *Genetics of Human Cancer,* Mulvihill, J. J., Miller, R. W., and Fraumeni, J. F., Eds., Raven Press, New York, 321.
37. **Pellegris, G., Illeni, M. T., Vaglini, M., Rovini, D., Cascinelli, N., and Masserini, C.,** HLA antigens in malignant melanoma patients, *Tumori,* 66, 51, 1980.
38. **Pollack, M. S. and Livingstone, P. O.,** HLA and DR antigen frequencies in melanoma patients: possible relation to disease prognosis, *Tissue Antigens,* 26, 262, 1985.
39. **Lamm, L. U., Kissmeyer-Nielsen, F., Kjerbye, K. E., Mogensen, B., and Petersen, N. C.,** HL-A and ABO antigens and malignant melanoma, *Cancer,* 33, 1458, 1974.
40. **Cavelier, B., Daveau, M., Gilbert, D., Fontaine, M., Cesarini, J. P., and Delpech, B.,** Augmentation de l'antigène HLA-A9 dans les mélanomes malins, principalement dans les formes métastatiques ou les récidives. A propos de 105 mélanomes dont 34 formes graves, *C.R. Acad. Sci. Paris,* 291, 241, 1980.
41. **Bergholtz, B., Brennhovd, I., Klepp, O., Kaakinen, A., and Thorsby, E.,** HLA antigens in malignant melanoma, *Cancer,* 39, 2342, 1977.
42. **Nathanson, S. D., Park, M. S., Drew, I., Morton, D. L., and Terasaki, P. I.,** Serologically defined B-lymphocyte antigen expression in patients with malignant melanoma, *Surg. Forum.,* 30, 147, 1979.
43. **Nathanson, S. D., Park, M. S., Drew, S. I., Morton, D. L., and Terasaki, P. I.,** First and second B-lymphocyte antigen expression in malignant melanoma, *Transplant. Proc.,* 12, 118, 1980.
44. **Barger, B. O., Acton, R. T., Soong, S. J., Roseman, J., and Balch, C.,** Increase of HLA-DR4 in melanoma patients from Alabama, *Cancer Res.,* 42, 4276, 1982.
45. **Mueller-Eckhardt, G., Schendel, D. J., Hundeiker, M., Riedel, R., O'Neill, G. J., Riethmuller, G., and Mueller-Eckhardt, C.,** Possible association between HLA-DR5 and superficial spreading melanoma (SSM), *Int. J. Cancer,* 34, 751, 1984.
46. **Wallace, D. G., Exton, L. A., and McLeod, G. R. C.,** Genetic factor in malignant melanoma, *Cancer,* 27, 1262, 1971.
47. **Duggleby, W. F., Stoll, H., Priore, R., Greenwald, P., and Graham, S.,** A genetic analysis of melanoma-polygenic inheritance as a threshold trait, *Am. J. Epidemiol.,* 114, 63, 1981.
48. **Anderson, D. E.,** Clinical characteristics of the genetic variety of cutaneous malignant melanoma in man, *Cancer,* 28, 7721, 1971.
49. **Lynch, H. T. and Krush, A. J.,** Heredity and malignant melanoma: implications for early cancer detection, *Can. Med. Assoc. J.,* 99, 17, 1968.
50. **Lynch, H. T., Fusaro, R. M., Pester, J., and Lynch, J. F.,** Familial atypical multiple mole-melanoma (FAMMM) syndrome: genetic heterogeneity and malignant melanoma, *Br. J. Cancer,* 42, 58, 1980.
51. **Lynch, H. T., Fusaro, R. M., Kimberling, W. J., Lynch, J. F., and Danes, B. S.,** Familial atypical multiple mole-melanoma (FAMMM) syndrome: segregation analysis, *J. Med. Genet.,* 20, 342, 1983.
52. **Elder, D. E., Goldman, L. I., Goldman, S. C., Greene, M. H., and Clark, W. H., Jr.,** Dysplastic nevus syndrome: a phenotypic association of sporadic cutaneous melanoma, *Cancer,* 46, 1787, 1980.
53. **Rahbari, H. and Mehregan, A. H.,** Sporadic atypical mole syndrome, *Arch. Dermatol.,* 117, 329, 1981.
54. **Crutcher, W. A. and Sagebiel, R. W.,** Prevalence of dysplastic naevi in a community practice, *Lancet,* 1, 729, 1984.
55. **Happle, R., Traupe, H., Vakilzadeh, F., and Macher, E.,** Arguments in favor of a polygenic inheritance of precursor nevi, *J. Am. Acad. Dermatol.,* 6, 540, 1982.
56. **Elston, R. C. and Stewart, J.,** A general model for the analysis of pedigree data, *Hum. Hered.,* 21, 523, 1971.
57. **Bale, S. J., Chakravarti, A., and Greene, M. H.,** Cutaneous malignant melanoma and familial dysplastic nevi: evidence for autosomal dominance and pleiotropy, *Am. J. Hum. Genet.,* 38, 188, 1986.
58. **Chase, G. A., Foldstein, M. F., Breitner, J. C., Beaty, T. H., and Self, S. G.,** The use of life tables and survival analysis in testing genetic hypotheses, with an application to Alzheimer's disease, *Am. J. Epidemiol.,* 117, 590, 1983.
59. **Avril, M. F.,** personal communication, 1987.
60. **Bergman, W., Palan, A., and Went, L. N.,** Clinical and genetic studies in six Dutch kindreds with the dysplastic naevus syndrome, *Ann. Hum. Genet.,* 50, 249, 1986.
61. **Hawkins, B. R., Dawkins, R. L., Hockey, A., Houliston, J. B., and Kirk, R. L.,** Evidence for linkage between HLA and malignant melanoma, *Tissue Antigens,* 17, 540, 1981.
62. **Hors, J., Demenais, F., Cesarini, J. P., Verola, O., Prade, M., Mueller-Eckhardt, G., Gazit, E., Gebuhrer, L., Busson, M., and Dawkins, R. L.,** HLA and familial malignant melanoma, in *Histocompatibility Testing* 1984, Albert, E. D., Baur, M. P., and Mayr, W. R., Eds., Springer-Verlag, Heidelberg, 1984, 407.
63. **Demenais, F., Cesarini, J. P., Daveau, M., Cavelier, B., Gony, J., Feingold, N., and Hors, J.,** A linkage study between HLA and cutaneous malignant melanoma or precursor lesions or both, *J. Med. Genet.,* 21, 429, 1984.

64. **Bale, S. J., Greene, M. H., Murray, C., Goldin, L. R., Johnson, A. H., and Mann, D.,** Hereditary malignant melanoma is not linked to the HLA complex on chromosome 6, *Int. J. Cancer,* 36, 439, 1985.
65. **Pellegris, G., Illeni, M. T., Rovini, D., Vaglini, M., Cascinelli, N., and Ghidoni, A.,** HLA complex and familial malignant melanoma, *Int. J. Cancer,* 29, 621, 1982.
66. **Demenais, F., Cesarini, J. P., and Hors, J.,** Study of the familial cosegregation of cutaneous malignant melanoma and/or precursor lesions and the HLA system, in *Familial Cancer,* Muller and Weber, Eds., S. Karger, Basel, 1985, 133.
67. **Hors, J., Gony, J. M., Andrieu, J. M., Cesarini, J. P., Teillet, F., Demenais, F., Feingold, N., Leverger, G., and Schaison, G.,** Participation of the major histocompatibility complex in the determination of familial malignancies, in *Familial Cancer,* Muller and Weber, Eds., S. Karger, Basel, 1985, 213.

Chapter 7

MOLECULAR GENETIC ANALYSES OF FUNCTIONAL MELANOMA-ASSOCIATED ANTIGENS

Lloyd H. Graf, Jr. and Soldano Ferrone

TABLE OF CONTENTS

I. INTRODUCTION

Immunological analyses of human melanoma cells have added significantly to the biological understanding of this severe form of cancer, and they have aided in developing diagnostic and therapeutic methods to combat it. Initiated, in part, in recognition of the autologous immunogenicity of many melanoma lesions, and of the implicit role of host immune responses in mediating the relatively frequent spontaneous regressions of melanoma,[1,2] studies employing immunological approaches have progressed at an accelerated pace since the advent of murine and human monoclonal antibody (mAb) technologies.

Comparative structural characterization of membrane-bound molecules detected by murine and human mAbs against melanoma cells has led to the definition of more than of 25 melanoma-asociated antigens (MAA) expressed by sporadic and familial melanoma cells.[3-5] Some of these are of interest for their potential utility as "targets" for immunodiagnostic or immunotherapeutic intervention, for functions or roles of possible significance to melanocytic neoplasia, or for insights that they may provide about cell surface correlates of oncogenesis, progression, or differentiation.[4]

Recently, immunochemical approaches to the characterization of several MAAs have been complemented by molecular analysis of recombinant clones for genes encoding their protein backbones. The isolation of such MAA gene recombinants has been made possible in large degree by the increasing practicability of several cloning approaches. These include DNA-mediated gene transfer of MAA-positive phenotypes, use of polysome immunoprecipitation and "subtraction" strategies to enrich for mRNAs or cDNAs of interest, use of cloning vectors that express cDNA inserts, and use of immunological library-screening methods.

Recombinant clones represent a source of structural insights about antigens, since primary amino acid sequences can be predicted from clonal DNA sequences. This approach is often more experimentally tenable than purifying and sequencing the protein molecules themselves. The inferred amino acid sequences can lead through computer-assisted modeling to the assignment of structural domains, the prediction of membrane and/or cytoskeleton association points, glycosylation patterns, lipid substitution or phosphorylation target sites, and other features. Comparative DNA sequence analyses can aid in detecting gene-associated cis-acting sequences for action of regulatory molecules mediating cytokine or other chemical responses, or cell type specificity of expression. RNA analyses using gene probes can elucidate transcriptional aspects of regulated antigen expression. DNA sequence comparisons can aid in identification of potential roles for the antigens as predicted by their resemblances to characterized receptors for growth factors, hormones, viruses, or nutrients; to matrix binding or cell adhesion molecules; or to membrane-associated enzymes. Punctuation patterns and chromosomal linkages of genomic genes, determined by use of cDNA probes in Southern and/or *in situ* chromosomal hybridization studies can support the identification of antigen "domains" and the detection of possible cytogenetic correlates of cancer-related antigen expression. Expression vectors can be used for reverse genetic dissection of cell specificity of antigen expression and for microbial production of large amounts of protoantigenic peptides. In the case of MAA and other tumor-associated antigens, the knowledge and constructs resulting from molecular approaches have begun to be employed for the design of promising immunotherapeutic strategies.

Genes specifying a number of MAAs have been isolated. These include "p97",[6] 96 kDa MAA/gp89/intercellular adhesion molecule-1 (ICAM-1),[7-10] nerve growth factor receptor (NGFR),[11] and two closely related glycoproteins detected by the mAb MUC18.[12] Recombinant genomic clones related to the gene for the melanoma-carcinoma associated antigen 100 kDa MAA have also been isolated.[13] Other MAAs have been found to be isogenic with antigens independently cloned as immune cells or other independently identified antigens;

these include HLA Class II antigens, the lymphocyte homing receptor CDw 44, and the Thy-1 glycoprotein.[14-21]

This review will describe the recombinant cloning of genes for the 96 kDa MAA/gp89/ICAM-1 molecule and for the p97 ("melanotransferrin") molecule. Cloning methods employed will be discussed, as representing general strategies available for loci having antigenic products. Structural, regulatory, and functional information gained through clonal analysis will be discussed as will possible recombinant-based strategies for clinical exploitation of these prototypical MAA.

II. 96 kDa MAA = gp89 = ICAM-1

The 96 kDa MAA is a membrane-bound glycoprotein that was identified by the mAbs, CL203, and CL207 raised against immune interferon gamma (IFN-γ)-treated human melanoma cells.[22] The mature 96 kDa MAA, as synthesized by human melanoma cells, has an apparent M_r of 96 kDa[22] to 89 kDa[23] as determined by SDS-PAGE. It is a "progression marker" for melanocytic lesions in that it is expressed by the great majority ($\geq$90%) of metastatic melanomas, by ~50% of primary melanomas (including particularly cells of potentially virulent vertical growth phase primary lesions), and by ~10% of nevi, while not being readily detected on normal melanocytes.[22,23] Synthesis of this molecule by melanoma and endothelial cells is enhanced, and synthesis by cells of certain other tumors and normal tissues is induced by treatment with IFN-γ, with tumor necrosis factor alpha (TNF-α), with tumor-promoting phorbol esters, with interleukin-1, with bacterial lipopolysaccharide, or with lymphotoxin.[22,24]

III. CELL ADHESION FUNCTION OF 96 kDa MAA

The 96 kDa MAA has recently been shown to have an adhesion function of possible significance to the pathogenesis of melanoma. Gene-level characterization and immunological specificity studies have shown that the 96 kDa MAA, the independently defined melanoma antigen gp89, defined by mAb 3.58,[23] the intercellular adhesion molecule ICAM-1 (CD54) defined by a variety of mAb including RR-1,[25] and the major rhinovirus receptor[26,27] are all isogenic species having essential structural identity to each other.

The ICAM-1 molecule has been observed to recognize and adhere to the leukocyte function antigen LFA-1, which is displayed in varying amounts by most leukocytic cells.[25] ICAM-1 also interacts with the adhesion molecule Mac-1, a LFA-1-related molecule that, like LFA-1, is a member of the integrin family of adhesion molecules.[28] These interactions lead to immunologically critical binding of ICAM-1- or Mac-1-positive cells to LFA-1-positive cells. ICAM-1, as expressed both by classical monocytic antigen-presenting cells such as macrophages and by epidermal keratinocytes, is known or suspected to amplify the histocompatibility antigen-dependent cell recognition events critical for systemic or local T-cell activation.[29] The ICAM-1:LFA-1 (Mac-1) interaction appears also to be important for granulocyte/neutrophil recruitment and retention phases of inflammatory responses such as those involved in allotypic graft rejection.[30]

The ICAM-1 gene product, as expressed by human melanoma cells and by transfected mouse melanoma cells, appears also to be capable of mediating adhesions with LFA-1$^+$ lymphocytes and lymphocytic cell lines.[31] It is hypothesized that these interactions may facilitate the formation by melanoma cells, of circulating "microemboli" with adherent leukocytes, and that these may have an advantage in terms of metastatic dissemination.[9] It is also reasonable to hypothesize that the presence of the functional 96 kDa MAA/ICAM-1 molecule on the surfaces of melanoma cells might lead to their disruption of normal cutaneous immune processes, thus facilitating survival of melanoma lesions. Whereas melanoma ICAM-1 could act as an attractant to augment epidermal recruitment of immune cells from the dermal circulation, the melanoma cells, which often co-express ICAM-1 and HLA Class II molecules, might then deficiently present as yet unidentified antigens to autologous helper T cells with immunosuppressive consequences.

IV. CLONING APPROACHES

Independent efforts by four laboratories have led to the isolation of cDNA clones that correspond to the gp89 and 96 kDa MAA as produced by human melanoma cells and by transfected mouse melanoma cells, respectively;[9,10] the ICAM-1 molecule as produced by endothelial cells and promyelocytic leukemia cells;[7,8] and major rhinovirus receptor as produced by human cervical carcinoma (HELA) cells.[26,27] Recently, a genomic clone containing a significant portion of the chromosomal ICAM-1 gene has also been isolated.[47] Currently effective strategies for isolating genes that specify immunologically identifiable molecules are well represented among the several antibody-assisted approaches that have been utilized to obtain these recombinant clones.

Staunton and co-workers[7] purified ICAM-1 from leukemic spleen cells by immunoaffinity chromatography using the anti-ICAM-1 mAb RR1/1. They then designed two oligonucleotides corresponding to portions of the ICAM-1 coding region as predicted from tryptic peptide amino acid sequences. Use of these oligonucleotides to probe cDNA libraries, one from phorbol ester-induced promyelocytic leukemia cells and the other from lipopolysaccharide-treated endothelial cells, yielded 12 cross hybridizable cDNA clones. Sequence information from representative clones predicted their specification of peptides identical to the characterized ICAM-1-derived peptides, confirming the homology of the clones to human ICAM-1 genes.

Johnson and co-workers[9] analyzed a cDNA library from IFN-γ stimulated human melanoma cells. The library was constructed in a cloning vector that directs metabolically inducible microbial expression of the cloned gene. They screened the library using four anti-gp89 mAbs, thus detecting a clone that synthesized an antibody-reactive product. Clone DNA sequence analyses and immunological cross reactivity studies demonstrated isogenicity of gp89 with ICAM-1.

Simmons, Makgoba, and Seed[8] used a cloning vector that directs mammalian cell expression of cloned sequences to construct a cDNA library from RNA of phorbol ester-induced human promyelocytic leukemia cells. They then screened clones from this library by ''panning'',[10] after introducing the clones into primate (COS) host cells, thus detecting clones that direct synthesis of surface antigens reactive with the anti-ICAM-1 mAbs 8F5 and 84H10.

Graf and co-workers[32] have employed an approach that involves DNA-mediated gene transfer to assist in identification of cDNA and genomic clones having homology to the 96 kDa MAA (=ICAM-1) gene. Total chromosomal DNA from human melanoma cells was applied as a calcium phosphate co-precipitate for primary 1° transfection of a gene encoding a mAb CL-203- reactive (96 kDa MAA-like) cell surface molecule into the highly-competent mouse melanoma host cell line B78H1. Secondary 2° and 3° transfections of the gene were carried out, using DNAs from the 1° and 2° transfectant cells, in order to delete from the genomes of transfectant cells, unselected human sequences not related to the 96 kDa MAA gene. At the stage of 3° transfection a ''selective co-amplification'' strategy was applied. These procedures, which are described in detail in Reference 32 and reviewed in References 4 and 31, led ultimately to the isolation of ''co-amplified'' 3° mouse melanoma transfectant cells that contain some 50 to 100 copies of the introduced human 96 kDa MAA gene and that express commensurately high levels (10^7 CL 203 binding sites/cell) of its antigenic product.

A cDNA library was constructed from polyadenylated RNA of the co-amplified transfectant cells in a bacteriophage vector. In recognition of the possible homology of 96 kDa MAA with ICAM-1, the cDNA library was screened with an ICAM-1 cDNA clone (kindly provided by Dr. D. Staunton, Center for Blood Research, Harvard Medical School, Boston, MA). Almost 1% of the clones were ICAM-1 homologous, an indication of the high concentration of gene transcripts in the transfectant cells. Four cDNA clones, having inserts ranging from 1.1 to ≥1.7 kb were clonally purified. The insert of one of these (1.65 kb) has been shown to encompass approximately 80% of the ICAM-1 protein coding region and to have essential restriction map and sequence identity to the ICAM-1 gene over this region.[10]

Recently a clone-containing chromosomal sequence homologous to a 5′-oriented 96 kDa/ICAM-1 cDNA clone has been isolated from a library of partially MboI-digested transfectant cell genomic DNA fragments by nucleic acid hybridization with one of our cDNA clones.[47] The sequences hybridizable with this cDNA clone (which corresponds to bp 260—1600 of ICAM-1 cDNA[7]) have been localized to a 2.5 to 3 kb restriction fragment within the 20 kb insert of the genomic clone, suggesting the possibility that the insert might contain flanking sequences, including cis-acting sites critical for regulated expression of the transfected gene, in addition to the detected coding sequences.

A. GENERAL APPLICABILITY OF CLONING APPROACHES

The cloning approaches described previously can be applied with varying degrees of generality as means of addressing the molecular cloning of immunologically defined molecules. For example, successful use of expression-based cDNA cloning strategies relies on the ability of antibodies to recognize unglycosylated microbial translation products; animal cell cDNA expression cloning relies on the nonexpression by host COS cells, of primate antigen homologs immunologically cross-reactive with the human antigen of interest; and transfection-based approaches can succeed only if the epitope(s) that react with the available antibodies are products of single genes of transfectable (≤50 kb) size. While the 96 kDa MAA/ICAM-1 molecule may be unusual in meeting all of these criteria, it is probable that the gene(s) encoding any given antigen will be subject to isolation by one or more of the approaches.

B. STRUCTURAL FEATURES OF 96 kDa MAA/ICAM-1 AS DEDUCED FROM GENE SEQUENCE

Comparative DNA sequence analyses have established that the 96 kDa MAA/ICAM-1 gene product is a member of the immunoglobulin superfamily, having 5 tandem extracellular domains homologous to immunoglobulin C2 constant-region-like chains. In this resemblance to immunoglobin molecules 96 kDa MAA/ICAM-1 is analogous to a number of membrane-bound virus receptors and adhesion molecules.[33] The 96 kDa MAA/ICAM-1 molecule is especially closely related to the nerve cell adhesion molecule N-CAM and to the myelin-associated glycoprotein.[7,8]

These deduced structural features and a reverse genetic approach have helped to elucidate the structural basis for the immunologically critical heterotypic binding of ICAM-1 with LFA-1.[34] Electron microscopic visualization of a genetically engineered soluble form of ICAM-1 lacking the cytoplasmic "tail" domain indicated that the 5 immunoglobulin-like regions of the molecule are aligned in an end-to-end succession forming a flexible rodlike configuration that can be linear or bent. The binding sites for antibodies that block ICAM-1 adhesion to LFA-1 were localized to the two domains most distal to the membranes (the N-terminal domains D1 and D2) by *in vitro* domain exchange experiments in which chimeric cDNA clones containing mixtures of human and murine ICAM-1 cDNAs were introduced into primate host cells. Reverse genetic analyses of *in vitro* mutagenized forms of human ICAM-1 cDNA indicated that several amino acid residues scattered through the extracellular portion of the most extracellular domains D1 and D2 are critical for LFA-1 binding. Groupings of residues such as RGEDE and PERVE, which had been considered to be possible LFA-1 contacting residues in view of the absence from ICAM-1 of the RGD grouping found to be important for many cell adhesion events, appear not to be critical.[34]

These studies are indicative of the way in which recombinant technology can be used to delineate the geometry and dissect structure-function relationships for the products of genes which have been cloned.

C. FUNCTION AND ROLE OF ICAM-1 EXPRESSED BY MELANOMA CELLS

Mammalian-expression vector-encoded ICAM-1 molecules[8] have been shown to have ICAM-1-like immunological activity when they are expressed by transfected mouse fibroblasts: the combined transgenomic expression of HLA Class II antigens and ICAM-1 molecules by fibroblasts enables them to function as antigen-presenting cells in the antigen-dependent mitogenic activation of T cells.[35]

It has been hypothesized (see Section III) that the adhesion capability of ICAM-1 may facilitate the progression or the metastatic spread of melanoma cells and that this functional contribution may provide a selective advantage *in vivo,* leading to enhanced ICAM-1 expression on cells of virulent primary or metastatic lesions.[9] Use of transfectable vectors to manipulate ICAM-1 expression by melanocytic cells at different stages of proliferative normalcy or neoplasia will assist in the testing of this hypothesis.

In addition, the development of transfectable cDNA clones specifying the active murine homologue of ICAM-1, ''MALA-2''[36-38] will permit testing of the importance of expression of functional ICAM-1 to mouse melanoma cell colonization and metastasis in defined syngeneic animal tumor models.

D. PROSPECTIVE APPLICATION OF 96 kDa MAA/ICAM-1 RECOMBINANTS

The 96 kDa MAA/ICAM-1 molecule of human carcinoma cells has been successfully targeted, using daunomycin-conjugated anti-96 kDa MAA mAb CL 207, to retard lesion formation in nude mice.[39] While the critical nature of ICAM-1 function in normal immune responses appears to be a complicating factor for ICAM-1-targeted treatment of human cancers, it is likely that availability of large amounts of the 96 kDa MAA/ICAM-1 gene product as synthesized by recombinant microorganisms will accelerate the fine structural immunological characterization of ICAM-1. The extracellular domains preferentially exposed on the post-translationally modified form(s) of the antigens produced by melanoma cells as compared to highly positive normal cells such as macrophages, Langerhans' cells, lymphocytes, and endothelial cells might then be identified and exploited.

Thus the cloning of the 96 kDa MAA/gp89/ICAM-1 gene may lead to advances in the understanding of the role of this glycoprotein in cancer progression and could facilitate the clinical utilization of the melanoma form of the molecule.

E. CLONING OF THE GENE SPECIFYING THE p97MAA AND DEVELOPMENT OF AN ANTI-p97 VACCINE

The transmembrane glycoprotein p97 (gp95,gp87) has been independently identified by mAbs raised by several groups.[40-42] It is present on most primary and metastatic melanomas, melanocytic nevi, and carcinomas in sweat glands and in fetal intestine, but it is expressed only in ''trace'' amounts on melanocytes and other normal adult tissues.

This distribution has fostered interest in p97 as a possible focus of active or passive immunotherapeutic approaches to melanoma. p97 derives further interest from its protein sequence homology to that of the iron-binding serum protein transferrin and from the transferrin-like ability of the p97 molecule to bind iron.[43] This function, which had led to the use of the name ''melanotransferrin'' for p97, is suggestive of a possible nutritional/metabolic role for the antigen in melanocytic neoplasia.

Recombinant clones for the p97 gene have been isolated, and their analysis has augmented understanding of the antigen's relationship to other members of the transferrin gene family. Moreover, a viral p97 gene expression vector is being tested as a possible vaccine for active stimulation of p97-targeted cellular and humoral immune responses.

F. CLONING OF p97 cDNAs

The strategy for cloning a p97 cDNA used a polysome immunoprecipitation (or immunochromatography) step to achieve 100- to 200(180)-fold purification of human melanoma messenger RNAs that were in the process of directing synthesis of nascent p97 peptide chains.[6] Screening of a cDNA library synthesized from this enriched mRNA fraction led to detection of a clone that preferentially hybridized the p97-enriched mRNA. Use of this cDNA clone, which was found to correspond to the 3′ end of the p97 gene, led to identification of additional p97 cDNA clones which collectively encompass the entire transcribed portion of the gene, and to the isolation of genomic clones.[44]

V. DEDUCED STRUCTURE AND FUNCTION OF THE p97 MOLECULE

DNA sequence analyses provided further support to the close homology of p97 to transferrin, and to other members of the transferrin supergene family including lactotransferrin and ovotransferrin. The predicted structure of p97 consists mainly of two 340—350 amino acid extracellular domains which have extensive homology both to each other and to previously characterized proteins of the transferrin family. The relative positioning of amino acids that form the putative binding pocket for iron and of disulfide bonds that interconnect the different domains are conserved in p97 as compared to other transferrins. The p97 gene is located on the long arm of chromosome 3, in close linkage to the genes for transferrin and for transferrin receptor.

It is hypothesized that the p97 gene was derived from the 30 to 40% homologous serum transferrin gene by a tandem gene duplication some 300 million years ago. A second tandem duplication is thought to have occurred at a later time, thus yielding the two extracellular p97 domains, which have 50% of their amino acid sequences in common.[44] The precise role of the metal-binding activity of this melanotransferrin molecule in tumor physiology remains to be determined.

VI. AN APPROACH TO ACTIVE IMMUNOTHERAPY EMPLOYING THE p97 GENE

A novel p97-directed antitumor vaccination strategy, which employs a recombinant vaccinia virus-p97 expression construct, has recently been tested in experimental animals. In the recombinant virus, a composite of p97 amino acid coding and punctuation sequence derived from cDNA and genomic clones was inserted into the vaccinia virus genome, so that this expression is directed by the viral "7.5 K" or thymidine kinase gene promoter.

Cells infected *in vitro* with this chronic virus, "v-p97NY", express copious amounts of a virus-encoded surface glycoprotein that is experimentally indistinguishable from native p97.[45,46]

The capacity of the v-p97NY virus to stimulate active anti-p97 immune responses was tested in mice and in macaque monkeys. The virus was introduced into these animals by tail scarification, a method presumably leading to the productive infection of body cells encountered by the introduced virus. Neither the mice nor the monkeys exhibited adverse effects from the inoculations. In both species v-p97NY exposure elicited humoral immune responses to p97. Unlike monkeys that had been immunized with purified p97, the virus-challenged monkeys also exhibited p97-dependent T-cell proliferation and delayed-type hypersensitivity responses. The mice that had been exposed to v-p97NY developed an enhanced ability to prevent pulmonary colonization by syngeneic mouse melanoma cells expressing human p97 from a transfected cDNA expression vector. The inoculated mice also had increased p97-targeted resistance to intravenous challenge with these cells. Treatment with v-p97NY virus also assisted mice in resisting tumors of human p97-positive mouse melanoma cells that had been administered 2 days prior to viral "immunizations".[46]

These results suggested the possible superiority of p97-specifying viruses to soluble p97 as inocula for the generation of active cellular immune responses targeted to antigen-positive cells. Clinical trials which are in a planning stage will assess the usefulness of v-p97NY to implement active specific immunotherapy in patients with melanoma.

In principle, similar viral vectors containing the genes specifying other cloned melanoma or tumor-associated antigens, such as NGFR, cDW44, Thy-1, 96 kDa MAA/ICAM-1, HLA Class II antigens, and others, can be constructed. It is conceivable that multideterminant vaccines involving mixtures of viruses will have value for the future active immunotherapy of melanoma.

VII. FUTURE PROSPECTS

Numerous glycoprotein and proteoglycan MAA have clinical and/or tumor biological interest comparable to those of the 96 kDa MAA/ICAM-1 and the p97 molecules. The molecular understanding of these MAA continues to advance as a growing number of the genes specifying them are being cloned by use of approaches including those outlined earlier. It is possible to envision a time in the relatively near future, when essentially all immunologically defined proteins preferentially synthesized by melanoma cells are accessible to gene level analysis. The resultant wealth of information about structures, regulated expression, neoplasia-related functions, and roles of the MAA genes and products will lead to a comprehensive topological view of the melanoma cell. This in turn will aid basic scientists and clinicians in their efforts to understand and to exploit the surface biology of malignant melanocytes.

REFERENCES

1. **Ferrone, A. and Pellegrino, M.,** Serological detection of human melanoma-associated antigens, in *Immunodiagnosis,* Herberman, R. B. and McIntyre, R., Eds., Marcel Dekker, New York, 1979, 588.
2. **Stuhlmiller, G. M.,** Immunobiology of melanoma, in *Clinical Management of Melanoma,* Seigler, H. F., Ed., Martinus Nijhoff Publishers, Boston, 1982, 233.
3. **Lloyd, K. O.,** Human tumor antigens: detection and characterization with monoclonal antibodies, in *Basic and Clinical Tumor Immunology,* Herberman, R. B., Ed., Martinus Nijhoff Publishers, Boston, 1983, 159.
4. **Graf, L. H., Jr. and Ferrone, S.,** Human melanoma-associated antigens, in *Human Immunogenetics,* Litwin, S. D., Ed., Marcel Dekker, New York, 1989, 643.
5. **Johnson, J. P., Stade, B. G., Rothbacher, U., Lehmann, J. M., and Riethmuller, G.,** Melanoma antigens and their association with malignant transformation and tumor progression, in *Human Melanoma. From Basic Research to Clinical Application,* Ferrone, S., Ed., Springer-Verlag, Heidelberg, 1990, 106.
6. **Rose, T. M., Plowman, G. D., Teplow, D. B., Dreyer, W. J., Hellstrom, K. E., and Brown, J. P.,** Primary structure of the human melanoma-associated antigen p97 (melanotransferrin) deduced from the mRNA sequence, *Proc. Natl. Acad. Sci. U.S.A.,* 83, 1261, 1983.
7. **Staunton, D. E., Marlin, S. D., Stratowa, C., Dustin, M. L., and Springer, T. A.,** Primary structure of ICAM-1 demonstrates interaction between members of the immunoglobulin and integrin supergene families, *Cell,* 52, 925, 1988.
8. **Simmons, D., Makgoba, M. W., and Seed, B.,** ICAM, an adhesion ligand of LFA-1, is homologous to the neural cell adhesion molecule NCAM, *Nature (London),* 331, 624, 1988.

9. **Johnson, J. P., Stade, B. G., Holzmann, B., Schwable, W., and Riethmuller, G.,** *De novo* expression of intercellular-adhesion molecule 1 in melanoma correlates with increased risk of metastasis, *Proc. Natl. Acad. Sci. U.S.A.*, 86, 641, 1986.
10. **Graf, L. H., Jr.,** Molecular cloning of genes that specify melanoma-associated antigens, in *Human Melanoma. From Basic Research to Clinical Application,* Ferrone, S., Ed., Spring-Verlag, Heidelberg, 1990.
11. **Chao, M. V., Bothwell, M. A., Ross, A. H., Koprowski, H., Lanahan, A. A., Buck, C. R., and Sehgal, A.,** Gene transfer and molecular cloning of the human NGF receptor, *Science,* 232, 518, 1986.
12. **Lehmann, J. M., Riethmuller, G., and Johnson, J. P.,** MUC18, a marker of tumor progression in human melanoma, shows sequence similarity to neural cell adhesion molecules of the immunoglobulin superfamily, *Proc. Natl. Acad. Sci. U.S.A.*, 86, 9891, 1989.
13. **Rosenberg, C. D., Ferrone, S., Hamby, C. V., Mancino, V., and Graf, L. H., Jr.,** Interspecific DNA-mediated transfer and amplification of a gene specifying a M_r 100,000 human melanoma-associated cell surface glycoprotein, *Cancer Res.*, 50, 1559, 1990.
14. **Natali, P. B., De Martino, C., Quaranta, V., Bigotti, A., Pellegrino, M. A., and Ferrone, S.,** Changes in Ia-like antigen expression on malignant human cells, *Immunogenetics,* 12, 409, 1981.
15. **Lee, J. S., Trowsdale, J., and Bodmer, W. F.,** cDNA clones coding for the heavy chain of human HLA-DR antigen, *Proc. Natl. Acad. Sci. U.S.A.*, 79, 545, 1982.
16. **Wake, C. T., Long, E. O., Strubin, M., Gross, N., Accolla, R., Carrel, S., and Mach, B.,** Isolation of cDNA clones encoding HLA-DR α chains, *Proc. Natl. Acad. Sci. U.S.A.*, 79, 6979, 1982.
17. **Hamby, C. V., et al,** in press, 1990.
18. **Stamenkovic, I., Amiot, M., Pesandro, J. M., and Seed, B.,** A lymphocyte molecule implicated in lymphnode homing is a member of the cartilage link protein family, *Cell,* 56, 1057, 1989.
19. **Goldstein, L. A., Zhou, D. F. H., Picker, L. J., Minty, C. N., Bargatze, R. F., Ding, J. F., and Butcher, E. C.,** A human lymphocyte homing receptor, the hermes antigen, is related to cartilage proteoglycan core and link proteins, *Cell,* 56, 1063, 1989.
20. **Hersey, P., Grace, J., Murray, E., Palmer, A., and McCarthy, W. H.,** Expression of Thy-1 antigen on human melanoma cells, *Int. J. Cancer,* 32, 21, 1983.
21. **Seki, T., Moriuchi, T., Chang, H. C., Denome, R., and Silver, J.,** Structural organization of the rat thy-1 gene, *Nature (London),* 313, 485, 1985.
22. **Matsui, M., Temponi, M., and Ferrone, S.,** Characterization of a monoclonal antibody-defined human melanoma-associated antigen susceptible to induction by immune interferon, *J. Immunol.*, 139, 2088, 1987.
23. **Holzmann, B., Johnson, J. P., Kaudewitz, P., and Riethmuller, G.,** In situ analysis of antigens on malignant and benign cells of the melanocyte lineage. Differential expression of two surface molecules, gp75 and gp89, *J. Exp. Med.*, 161, 366, 1985.
24. **Pober, J. S., Gimbrone, Jr., M. A., Lapierre, L. A., Mendrick, D. L., Fiers, W., Rothlein, R., and Springer, T. A.,** Overlapping patterns of activation of human endothelial cells by interleukin 1, tumor necrosis factor, and immune interferon, *J. Immunol.*, 137, 1893, 1986.
25. **Rothlein, R., Dustin, M. L., Marlin, S. D., and Springer, T. A.,** A human intercellular adhesion molecule (ICAM-1) distinct from LFA-1, *J. Immunol.*, 137, 1270, 1986.
26. **Greve, J. M., Davis, G., Meyer, A. M., Forte, C. P., Yost, S. C., Marlor, C. W., Kamarck, M. E., and McClelland, A.,** The major human rhinovirus receptor is ICAM-1, *Cell,* 56, 839, 1989.
27. **Staunton, D. E., Merluzzi, V. J., Rothlein, R., Barton, R., Marlin, S. D., and Springer, T. A.,** A cell adhesion molecule, ICAM-1, is the major surface receptor for rhinoviruses, *Cell,* 56, 849, 1989.
28. **Corbi, A. L., Kishimoto, T. K., Miller, L. J., and Springer, T. A.,** The human leukocyte adhesion glycoprotein Mac-1 (Complement receptor type 3, CD11b) α subunit: cloning, primary structure, and relation to the integrins, von Willebrand factor, and factor B, *J. Biol. Chem.*, 263, 12403, 1988.
29. **Nickoloff, B. J.,** Role of interferon-δ in cutaneous trafficking of lymphocytes with emphasis on molecular and cellular adhesion events, *Arch. Dermatol.*, 124, 1835, 1988.
30. **Kupper, T. S.,** Mechanisms of cutaneous inflammation. Interactions between epidermal cytokines, adhesion molecules, and leukocytes, *Arch. Dermatol.*, 125, 1406, 1989.
31. **Graf, L. H., Jr., Maier, G. D., and Schrementi, J. P.,** A transfected human melanoma-associated antigen expressed by mouse melanoma host cells mediates intra- and inter-specific leukocyte adhesion reactions, *J. Cell Biol.*, 109, 79 (Abstr.), 1989.
32. **Graf, L. H., Jr., Rosenberg, C. D., Mancino, V., and Ferrone, S.,** Transfer and co-amplification of a gene encoding a 96-kDa immune IFN-inducible human melanoma-associated antigen. Preferential expression by mouse melanoma host cells, *J. Immunol.*, 141, 1054, 1988.
33. **White, J. M. and Littman, D. R.,** Viral receptors of the immunoglobulin superfamily, *Cell,* 56, 725, 1989.
34. **Staunton, D. E., Dustin, M. L., Erickson, H. P., and Springer, T. A.,** The arrangement of the immunoglobulin-like domains of ICAM-1 and the binding sites for LFA-1 and rhinovirus, *Cell,* 61, 243, 1990.

35. **Altmann, D. M., Hogg, N., Trowsdale, J., and Wilkinson, D.,** Cotransfection of ICAM-1 and HLA-DR reconstitutes human antigen-presenting cell function in mouse L cells, *Nature (London),* 338, 512, 1989.
36. **Ballantyne, C. M., O'Brien, W. E., and Beaudet, A. L.,** Nucleotide sequence of the cDNA for murine intercellular adhesion molecule-1 (ICAM-1), *Nucleic Acid Res.,* 17, 5853, 1989.
37. **Siu, G., Hedrick, S. M., and Brian, A. A.,** Isolation of the murine intercellular adhesion molecule-1 (ICAM-1) gene. ICAM-1 enhances antigen-specific T-cell activation, *J. Immunol.,* 143, 3813, 1989.
38. **Horley, K. J., Carpenito, C., Baker, B., and Takei, F.,** Molecular cloning of murine intercellular adhesion molecule (ICAM-1), *EMBO J.,* 8, 2889, 1989.
39. **Matsui, M., Nakanishi, T., Noguchi, T., and Ferrone, S.,** Synergistic *in vitro* antitumor effect of daunomycin-anti-96-kDa melanoma-associated antigen monoclonal antibody CL 207 conjugate and recombinant IFN-γ, *J. Immunol.,* 141, 1410, 1988.
40. **Brown, J. P., Nishiyama, K., Hellstrom, I., and Hellstrom, K. E.,** Structural characterization of human melanoma-associated antigen p97 using monoclonal antibodies, *J. Immunol.,* 127, 539, 1981.
41. **Dippold, W. G., Lloyd, K. O., Li, L. T. C., Ikeda, H., Oettgen, H. F., and Old, L. J.,** Cell surface antigens of human malignant melanoma: definition of six antigenic systems with mouse monoclonal antibodies, *Proc. Natl. Acad. Sci. U.S.A.,* 77, 6114, 1980.
42. **Liao, S. K., Clarke, B. J., Khosravi, M., Kwong, P. C., Brickenden, A., and Dent, P. B.,** Human melanoma-specific oncofetal antigen defined by a mouse monoclonal antibody, *Int. J. Cancer,* 30, 573, 1982.
43. **Brown, J. P., Hewick, R. M., Hellstrom, I., Hellstrom, K. E., Doolittle, R. F., and Dreyer, W. J.,** Human melanoma-associated antigen p97 is structurally and functionally related to transferrin, *Nature (London),* 296, 171, 1982.
44. **Estin, C. D., Plowman, G. D., Rose, T. M., and Brown, J. P.,** Characterization of p97, a human melanoma-associated antigen, and development of a recombinant vaccine for melanoma, in *Human Melanoma. From Basic Research to Clinical Application,* Ferrone, S., Ed., Springer-Verlag, Heidelberg, 1990, 87.
45. **Hu, S.-L., Plowman, G. D., Sridhar, P., Stevenson, U. S., Brown, J. P., and Estin, C. D.,** Characterization of a recombinant vaccinia virus expressing human melanoma-associated antigen p97, *J. Virol.,* 62, 176, 1988.
46. **Estin, C. D., Stevenson, U. S., Plowman G. D., Hu, S.-L., Sridhar, P., Hellstrom, I., Brown, J. P., and Hellstrom, K. E.,** Recombinant vaccinia virus vaccine against the human melanoma antigen p97 for use in immunotherapy, *Proc. Natl. Acad. Sci. U.S.A.,* 85, 1052, 1988.
47. **Maier, G. D. and Graf, L. H., Jr.,** in preparation.

Chapter 8

EGF-RECEPTOR GENE, X-*src* ONCOGENE, AND INOSITOL LIPID TURNOVER IN KEY PROCESSES PRECEDING MELANOMA IN THE *XIPHOPHORUS* MODEL

A. D. Smith, Th. Gronau, A. Pröfrock, Ch. Zechel, I. M. Bird, P. A. Lane, A. Barnekow, and F. Anders

TABLE OF CONTENTS

I. INTRODUCTION

Wild populations of the fish genus *Xiphophorus* that inhabit fresh waters in Central America and their inbred descendants, are virtually insusceptible to all kinds of neoplasia, even when treated with carcinogens or tumor promoters. However, if hybrids are bred in the laboratory from crossings between different wild populations, some genotypes then are found to develop tumors after treatment with carcinogens. Other hybrid genotypes develop neoplasia after treatment with tumor promoters, while in a further group neoplasia develops spontaneously and is inherited in a Mendelian fashion.[3,11] This paper will concentrate on hereditary melanoma, the most prominent of the neoplasms that occur.

The melanomas grow out from black spots consisting of incompletely differentiated pigment cells[24] that are neoplastically transformed.[49] The spots can be assigned to certain black spot patterns which are apparent in the parental wild fish but do not grow out to become melanomas.[10]

II. GENETIC APPROACH

A. THE EXPERIMENTAL FISH

The fish used for the initial crosses in this work were females of *X. maculatus* (platyfish) derived from the wild population of Rio Jamapa, and males of *X. helleri* (swordtail) from Rio Lancetilla (see Plate 5, A and B*). The fish were collected by Myron Gordon[24] in 1939 and 1951, respectively, and have been inbred since that time. The platyfish (see Plate 5, A) exhibits a macromelanophore spot pattern, known as "spotted dorsal", which is confined to the dorsal fin; and a pterinophore pattern, "dorsal red", which is also confined to the dorsal fin but may extend, although weakly, to the adjoining parts of the body of the fish. In contrast, in the swordtail (see Plate 5, B) such pigment cell patterns have not evolved.

B. THE TUMOR GENE-COMPLEX (*Tu*)

The genes underlying the pigment cell patterns of the platyfish are located in a terminal Giemsa band of the X chromosome[1] and, based on 103 structural mutations,[4,52,53] can be roughly mapped as follows (commas represent the observed breaking points): *X . . . . .,Ptr, Df′, erbB*, Mel′-Tu.*

These genes represent a complex (*Tu*-complex) consisting of (1) the pterinophore locus (*Ptr*), which is responsible for pterinophore differentiation; (2) the compartment-specific dorsal fin locus *Df* which, in its mutated state, *Df′*, restricts the ability of both the pterinophore and macromelanophore to differentiate within the dorsal fin; (3) the region in which a viral *erb*B related oncogene (*erb*B*, i.e., a gene related to the receptor gene of the human epidermal growth factor, EGF) is located; (4) the melanophore locus *Mel* which, in its mutated state, *Mel′*, appears to allow *Df′* and *erb*B* directed pigment cell transformation; and (5) the arbitrarily symbolized "tumor gene" (*Tu*) which appears as a Mendelian factor but might be composed of both *erb*B* and *Mel*.

At least 20 linked genes are involved in the regulation of the *Tu*-complex, but there are also several nonlinked regulatory genes, e.g., the *Diff*-gene which, if present in the homozygous state, restrain the transformed pigment cells from proliferation by terminal differentiation.[5,6,10]

The *Tu*-complex of *X. maculatus* is "accessory" (i.e., not essential) to the fish. *X. helleri* has neither evolved a comparable *Tu*-complex nor the linked and nonlinked regulatory genes. In both, platyfish and swordtail, however, an "indispensable" *Tu*-complex was identified.[3,52] This *Tu*-complex is very difficult to deregulate and to trace by its tumorigenic potential, and is, therefore, not discussed here.

* Plate 5 appears following page 102.

C. THE *Tu*-COMPLEX IN CROSSINGS

1. Wild Platyfish × Wild Swordtail

When a *X. maculatus* female is crossed with a *X. helleri* male (see Plate 5, A and B), hybrids of the F_1 generation (C) all exhibit the "dorsal red" coloration which, however, is intensified and extended to the trunk of the fish, and all develop benign melanomas instead of the maternal spots. Backcrosses of the F_1 hybrids (C) with *X. helleri* (B) exhibit Mendelian segregation of the BC_1 hybrids, so that 25% develop benign melanomas on a reddish colored skin (D), 25% develop lethal malignant melanomas on the reddish skin (E), while 50% are grayish and, like *X. helleri,* they have no tumors or spots (F). For further backcrosses with the swordtail, BC hybrids bearing benign melanomas were used and the same segregation of the offspring was obtained.

Since platyfish and swordtails have a high number of chromosomes (n = 48) and since clear-cut information on the origin of their chromosomes was required to evaluate the experiments we planned, the experimental BC fish were taken from highly backcrossed generations ranging between BC_8 and BC_{22}. The genome of these hybrids consists virtually of swordtail chromosomes, except for the *Tu*-complex-containing X chromosome and the *Diff*-containing autosome that are selected by the crosses of the BC hybrids bearing benign melanomas and the swordtail (see Plate 5: D, E, and F). The phenotypic over-expression of the *Tu*-complex depends mainly on the replacement of platyfish autosomes carrying regulatory genes such as the differentiation gene *Diff*, by swordtail autosomes lacking such genes.[5]

2. Golden Platyfish × Golden Swordtail

We also included fish which were bred according to the procedure shown in Plate 5 but had a homozygous genetic block of pigment cell differentiation, namely, the "golden" block, *g/g*, that originated from the swordtail. The *g/g* condition prevents the development of spots and of melanomas. Alleviation of the block by tumor promoters such as 12-*o*-tetradecanoylphorbol-13-acetate (TPA), testosterone, and methylandrostenolone,[34] or a water extract of betel nuts[46] leads to a partial restoration of pigmentation, and to melanoma formation in the fish with genotypes corresponding to the melanomatous animals of Plate 5, D and E.[5,12,22,34,39,40]

3. Platyfish Mutants × Wild Swordtail

In addition to these genotypes, structural mutants were required for a more rigorous analysis of the processes preventing from or leading to neoplasia. Therefore, we selected X-ray-induced structurally mutated *Tu*-complexes of the platyfish,[4,52-54] bred them in platyfish strains, and introduced them (see Plate 5) by introgressive breeding into the genome of the swordtail. In particular (see Table 1), a mutant strain of *X. maculatus* was used that lacked the "spotted dorsal" pattern, but exhibited the "dorsal red" pattern. This genotype is referred to as *Ptr Df' erb*B*, indicating that the terminal *Mel'-Tu* chromosome region is deleted and that the break point is located between *erb*B* and *Mel'-Tu*. Backcross hybrids like those of the melanomatous segregants in the crossing scheme but carrying this deletion chromosome, are not susceptible to melanoma formation (see Plate 5, E). For comparison we used a phenotypically similar structural mutation, *Ptr Df'*, created by a different deletion event on a different break point so that *erb*B* *Mel'-Tu* is lost. The backcross hybrids carrying this deletion chromosome (E_2) are virtually indistinguishable by their reddish phenotype from those carrying the *Ptr Df' erb*B* chromosome. Another strain, designated "gray" *Df' erb*B* *Mel'-Tu*, carries a hybrid chromosome consisting of a swordtail autosome and the terminally translocated *Df' erb*B* *Mel'-Tu* platyfish chromosome fragment. The *Ptr* locus was lost during translocation of this hybrid chromosome. This translocation chromosome allows melanomas to form in the dorsal fin of the backcross hybrids which, because of the loss of the *Ptr* locus, lack the reddish coloration (E_3). Table 1 summarizes the phenotypic expression of the standard and mutated *Tu*-complexes in the platyfish and the swordtail genome.

TABLE 1
Phenotypic Expression of the Standard and Structurally Mutated *Tu*-Complexes in the Genome of Platyfish and Swordtail

Tu-complex	Denomination	Phenotype in the genome of: Platyfish	Swordtail
Ptr Df' erbB Mel'-Tu*	Standard	Dorsal red, spotted dorsal	Reddish, melanoma
Ptr Df' erbB,*	*Mel'-Tu* deletion	Dorsal red, no spots	Reddish, no melanoma
Ptr Df',	*erbB* Mel'-Tu* deletion	Dorsal red, no spots	Reddish, no melanoma
. . . ,Df' erbB Mel'-Tu*	Swordtail/platyfish translocation, *Ptr* deletion	No dorsal red, spotted dorsal	Gray, melanoma

Note: For symbols see legend of Plate 5.

III. MOLECULAR AND BIOCHEMICAL APPROACH

A. EXPRESSION OF x-*src* AND x-*erb*B* IN MELANOMA AND BRAIN

Molecular hybridization techniques, using c-DNA probes of retroviral oncogenes (v-*onc* genes) and DNA from normal tissues of *X. maculatus* and *X. helleri* revealed cellular counterparts (c-*onc* genes) of all 14 v-*onc* genes tested.[8,9] By immunoprecipitation[13,20] the xiphophorine counterpart of the Rous sarcoma virus oncogene product, pp60$^{x\text{-}src}$ kinase, was shown to be active in several healthy tissues of *Xiphophorus,* particularly in brain tissues.[41] In fish susceptible to melanoma caused by crossing, pp60$^{x\text{-}src}$ activity in the brain was three times higher than that of the insusceptible segregants, whereas the activity in the melanoma was elevated up to three times above that of the already elevated activity in the brain of the susceptible fish. Depending on the genetically determined degree of malignancy, the pp60$^{x\text{-}src}$ activity of a particular individual may be increased in parallel in both the melanoma and the brain[8,9,14,40,43] reflecting the neurogenic origin of the brain and of the pigment cell system. More recently, the activity of the xiphophorine *erb*B* (x-*erb*B*) located in the *Tu*-complex was found to correlate with *Tu*-complex expression in the melanoma, and in melanoma-derived cell line, somewhat more rigorously than was found for pp60$^{x\text{-}src}$.[52-54]

B. GROWTH REGULATION AND INOSITOL LIPID TURNOVER IN MELANOMAS

Recent interest in the possible involvement of phosphoinositide metabolism in growth regulation[15,38] raises the question of the status of the relevant enzymic pathways in the *Xiphophorus* genotypes. The need to investigate these enzyme systems was reinforced by the recent demonstration[21,27] that a potential substrate for pp60$^{c\text{-}src}$ kinase activity is phosphatidylinositol (PtdIns) kinase. One form of this enzyme initiates the pathway for the synthesis of the polyphosphoinositides. Some forms of PtdIns kinase bring about the phosphorylation of PtdIns to phosphatidylinositol 4-monophosphate (PtdIns4-P), which then can be phosphorylated to phosphatidylinositol 4,5-bisphosphate (PtdInsP_2). However, one form of the enzyme (type 1) is now known to phosphorylate PtdIns to PtdIns 3-P.[51] Phosphorylation of type 1 PtdIns kinase by pp60$^{c\text{-}src}$ activates the enzyme, enhancing formation of PtdInsP.[21,27]

A further connection between growth regulation and inositide metabolism arises from the demonstration that in some mammalian and human cell types, activation of the receptor for epidermal growth factor (EGF) enhances phosphoinositide metabolism.[25,35,50] These findings are of high interest with respect to melanoma formation in *Xiphophorus.* It was shown that the X-chromosomal x-*erb*B*, which is highly homologous to the human EGF receptor gene (*h-egfr*), could be involved in the first step leading to melanoma because it is part of the *Tu* gene complex.[52] Therefore, we were prompted to examine the activity of the enzymes

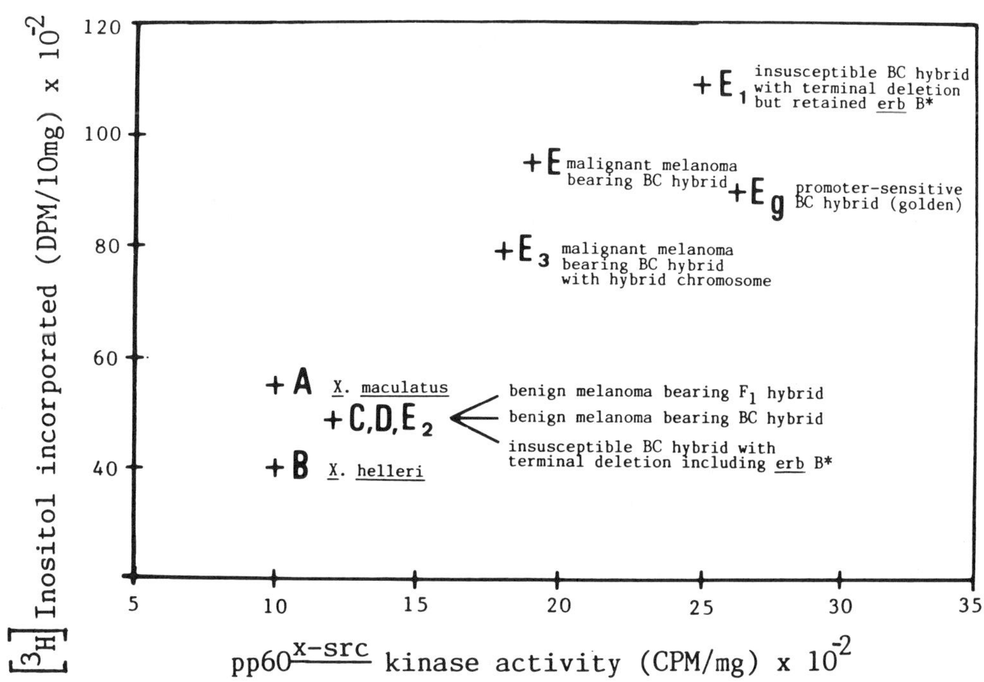

FIGURE 1. Incorporation of [^{3}H]inositol in phosphatidylinositol in brain extracts, plotted against activity of pp60$^{x\text{-}src}$ kinase. Capital letters represent the fish shown in Plate 5 and listed in Table 2. Note the correlation of both parameters.

arise as a result of a genotype-specific activation of PtdIns kinase by pp60$^{x\text{-}src}$ kinase, but such a correlation does not necessarily indicate a causal relationship. The recent demonstration[29,33,45] that the phospholipase C gene and the cellular *src* oncogene share sequences that lie in a putative regulatory domain suggests there may be alternative mechanisms involving a common activation step.

High levels of x-*src*-expression[43] and elevated phosphoinositide turnover[36] were found not only in the brain but also in all kinds of tumors of the fish tested. Other laboratories that studied the activities of c-*src* and PtdIns kinase in transformed cell lines in other organisms detected a similar parallelism.[21,23,27,47] However, to our knowledge, no one has described the highly complex result, that the healthy brain and the malignant neoplasm show elevated phosphoinositide turnover and cellular *src* expression, and that this correlation parallels the capacity of healthy fish to develop hereditary malignant tumors.

IV. PREDICTIONS ON MELANOMA FORMATION

We consistently found elevated phosphoinositide turnover and x-*src* kinase activity in the healthy brain before or after the onset of the malignant melanomas; therefore, these may serve as markers for malignant melanoma formation. Predictions can be made about whether a certain individual harboring the accessory *Tu*-complex is prone to develop malignant melanomas. In groups of genetically unknown individuals lacking or exhibiting spots or benign melanomas it is possible to discriminate between the animals that will not change and those that will proceed to lethal malignant melanomas. The type (E_1) BC hybrid that, in spite of its high phosphoinositide turnover, is incapable of developing melanomas, proves to be an exception, because target cells are lacking as a consequence of the *Mel'-Tu* deletion. The genetic changes underlying the malignant melanomas, i.e., the elimination and impairment of regulatory genes for the *Tu*-complex, have occurred in the germ cells of the preceding generations and operate in all somatic cells of the susceptible genotypes and their descendants, irrespective of whether cells capable of forming malignant melanomas are present. Therefore, the activities of the x-*src* and the phosphoinositide metabolic pathways are elevated in all tissues of the susceptible fish, including the brain and the melanoma.

In contrast, fish — for instance, type (A), (C), (D) — that require carcinogen-induced somatic mutations of particular regulatory genes of the *Tu*-complex for initiation of malignant melanomas, an infrequent tumor etiology discussed elsewhere,[3,8] show standard inositol incorporation and standard x-*src* activity in the brain (and the other tissues). Only malignant melanomas (and other neoplasms) induced in these genotypes show elevated inositol incorporation[36] and elevated x-*src* activity.[43] The malignant melanomas of these animals cannot be predicted by the inositol lipid turnover and $pp60^{x\text{-}src}$ kinase activity in healthy tissues.

V. REFLECTIONS ON KEY PROCESSES IN MELANOMA FORMATION OF *XIPHOPHORUS*

The results obtained with the BC_n hybrids carrying a complete or partially deleted *Tu*-complex require a more detailed discussion because they open up possibilities of intervention in key mechanisms critical to transformation and tumor induction. These BC_n hybrids were genetically identical, in as much as they were descended from wild populations, were inbred for 40 to 50 years, and were produced by crossings and consequent backcrossings. Their differences were in the structure (standard or deletion) of the *Tu*-complex — see Plate 5 (E, E_1, E_2, E_3) — and in pigment cell differentiation, which is arrested in the ''golden'' (*g/g*) animals (E_g). On the one hand, both the BC_n types (E) and (E_3) show a deregulation of the *Tu*-complex which is sufficient for spontaneous melanoma formation. The deficiency of the pterinophore locus *Ptr* and the pterinophores in the BC_n (E_3) animals has no detectable effect on melanoma development and melanoma growth, although pteridines are supposed to promote differentiation of transformed xiphophorine pigment cells *in vitro*.[30,37] Both $pp60^{x\text{-}src}$ kinase activity and phosphoinositide inositol turnover are elevated. On the other hand, the BC_n type (E_1) and the BC_n type (E_g) are protected from melanomas. The explanation appears to be simple, inasmuch as the type (E_1) BC_n animals lack the *Mel'-Tu* chromosome fragment that probably codes for the differentiation of cells that form the melanomas, whereas the (E_g) BC_n animals harbor a gene that retards the differentiation of these cells at the stem cell stage.[7] The oncostatic effect observed in both genotypes, therefore, is due to two different developmental factors that stop the appearance of those pigment cell precursors that form melanomas. The activity of the $pp60^{x\text{-}src}$ kinase and the phosphoinositide inositol turnover in the tumor-free BC_n animals of type (E_1) and type (E_g) are independent from melanomas suggesting that the molecular and biochemical machinery that is probably involved in melanoma formation may be running by genetic reasons without forming melanomas. Thus, it may be possible to uncouple mechanisms predisposed to melanomas from those mechanisms that realize the formation of melanomas. Although it was recently suggested[2] that alterations in inositol phospholipid metabolism in transformed cells may be regarded as a biochemical marker for neoplastic transformation, the distinction between predisposition and realization of neoplasia has not so far been possible in studies restricted to carcinogen-induced neoplasms. Our results indicate that there may be a particular type of activation of the cellular *src* gene and the genes of the inositol phospholipid system that is a marker for a predisposition to neoplasia, i.e., a pro-neoplastic condition.

VI. x-*erb*B* AS A CANDIDATE FOR AN INITIATOR OF INITIAL PROCESSES PRECEDING THE MORPHOLOGICAL REALIZATION OF MELANOMAS

Nothing is known about the key genes critical in starting the molecular and biochemical machinery before a tumor is initiated. Fortunately, from studies of platyfish- and swordtail-specific lengths of restriction fragments of xiphophorine oncogenes, we can discriminate the parental origin of a certain oncogene in a particular hybrid. In our highly backcrossed hybrids bearing malignant melanomas, the *Tu*-complex carrying X chromosome is the only chromosome that originates from the platyfish; 47 chromosomes originate from the swordtail. Out of 14 oncogenes studied only x-*erb*B* was inherited from the platyfish chromosome. Northern blots showed that the platyfish-derived x-*erb*B and several swordtail-derived oncogenes, including x-*src*, x-*erb*B, x-*sis*, x-*pdgf-r*, x-*ras*, x-*myc*, x-*myb*, and x-*erb*A are active in the melanoma.[31,32,44,54] The molecular and biochemical machinery which causes the development of the melanoma in the BC_n hybrid is, therefore, mainly run by swordtail-derived genes, while the signal for starting the machinery must be created and transmitted by a platyfish-derived gene. This gene must be located on the platyfish chromosome containing the *Tu*-complex which, in the present research, is an X chromosome. Among the oncogenes tested so far the x-*erb*B* gene, i.e., a gene related to the xiphophorine and human EGF-receptor gene, is the only one that is located in the chromosome region of the *Tu*-complex from which the signal for melanoma formation comes. The BC_n deletion mutant E_2 (see Plate 5, Figure 1, and Table 2) which appears to differ from the E_1 BC_n deletion mutant, only in lacking x-*erb*B*, indicates that both the $pp60^{x\text{-}src}$ activity and the phosphoinositide inositol turnover are resting at the normal level in the absence of x-*erb*B*. Our results thus indicate that the enhanced phosphoinositide turnover and the elevated $pp60^{c\text{-}src}$ activity that we observed is intimately coupled with the inheritance of x-*erb*B*, which presumably is involved in the key signal preceding melanoma formation in *Xiphophorus*.

VII. RECAPITULATION AND CONCLUSIONS

Certain backcross hybrids ($BC_{8\text{-}22}$) of *Xiphophorus maculatus* (platyfish) and *X. helleri* (swordtail; the recurrent parent), which carry a certain platyfish-derived chromosome among the swordtail chromosomes (2n = 48), may develop malignant melanomas caused by somatic mutation of a pigment cell precursor. The chromosome of the platyfish contains a tumor gene complex (*Tu*-complex) composed of a melanocyte determining gene (*Mel*), regulatory genes (*R*), and a v-*erb*B-related oncogene (x-*erb*B*). x-*erb*B* and swordtail-derived oncogenes are expressed in the melanoma, and phosphatidylinositol (PtdIns) turnover and $pp60^{x\text{-}src}$ kinase activity are elevated in the melanoma as compared to the healthy brain. Several germ line mutations opened up possibilities of intervention in key mechanisms critical to tumor development in the BC generations:

1. A mutant that lacks a *Tu*-complex-specific regulatory gene develops melanomas "spontaneously." PtdIns metabolism and x-*src* activity were not only enhanced in the melanomas but also in the healthy brain.
2. A mutant which is protected from spontaneous melanomas by an arrest of pigment cell differentiation showed high PtdIns turnover and x-*src* activity in the brain. Tumor promoters gave rise to melanomas which adopted the elevated PtdIns turnover and x-*src* activity of the brain.
3. A mutant that lacks *Mel* showed, although insusceptible to melanomas, the elevation of PtdIns turnover and x-*src* activity in the brain.

4. Another insusceptible mutant that lacks both *Mel* and x-*erb*B* showed a resting PtdIns turnover and a resting x-*src* activity in the brain.

We conclude that the signal for starting the molecular and biochemical machinery which initiates melanomas in the BC hybrids, and the enhanced PtdIns turnover and the elevated $pp60^{x\text{-}src}$ kinase activity that we observed are intimately coupled with the inheritance of x-*erb*B*, which presumably is involved in the key signal preceding melanomas in *Xiphophorus*.

ACKNOWLEDGMENTS

This work was supported by The Nuffield Foundation, EMBO, Umweltbundesamt, and Deutsche Forschungsgemeinschaft. We thank Dr. M. J. Berridge (Cambridge) for his helpful discussion and A. Woodhead (Brookhaven) for his critical reading of the manuscript.

REFERENCES

1. **Ahuja, M. R., Lepper, K., and Anders, F.,** Sex chromosome aberrations involving loss and translocation of tumor-inducing loci, in *Xiphophorus, Experientia,* 35, 28, 1979.
2. **Alonso, T., Morgan, R. O., Marvison, J. C., Zarbl, H., and Santos, E.,** Malignant transformation by *ras* and other oncogenes produces common alterations in inositol phospholipid signaling pathways, *Proc. Natl. Acad. Sci. U.S.A.,* 85, 4271, 1988.
3. **Anders, A. and Anders, F.,** Etiology of cancer as studied in the platyfish-swordtail system, *Biochem. Biophys. Acta,* 516, 61, 1978.
4. **Anders, A., Anders, F., and Klinke, K.,** Regulation of gene expression in the Gordon-Kosswig melanoma system I & II, in *Genetics and Mutagenesis of Fish,* Schröder, J. H., Ed., Springer-Verlag, New York, 1973, 33.
5. **Anders, A., Dess, G., Nishimura, S., and Kersten, H.,** A molecular approach to the study of malignancy and benignancy in melanoma of *Xiphophorus,* in *Pigm. Cell,* Bagnara, J., Klaus, S. N., Paul, E., and Schartl, M., Eds., University of Tokyo Press, Tokyo, 1985, 315.
6. **Anders, F.,** Tumor formation in platyfish-swordtail hybrids as a problem of gene regulation, *Experientia,* 23, 1, 1967.
7. **Anders, F.,** The biology of an oncogene, based upon studies on neoplasia in *Xiphophorus,* in *Biochemistry of Differentiation and Morphogenesis,* Jaenicke, L., Ed., Springer-Verlag, Berlin, 1982, 91.
8. **Anders, F.,** The Mildred Scheel memorial lecture — a biologist's view of human cancer, in *Modern Trends in Human Leukemia,* Vol. 8, Neth, R., Gallo, R. C., Greaves, M. F., Gaedicke, G., and Ritter, J., Eds., Springer-Verlag, Berlin, 1989, 23.
9. **Anders, F., Anders, A., Schartl, M., Gronau, T., Lüke, W., Schmidt, C.-R., and Barnekow, A.,** Oncogenes in development, neoplasia, and evolution, in *New Experimental Modalities in the Control of Neoplasia,* Chandra, P., Ed., Plenum Press, New York, 1987, 15.
10. **Anders, F., Diehl, H., and Scholl, E.,** Differentiation of normal melanophores and neoplastically transformed melanophores in the skin of fishes of genus *Xiphophorus,* in *The Skin of Vertebrates,* Spearman, R. I. C. and Riley, P. A., Eds., Academic Press, London, 1980, 211.
11. **Anders, F., Schartl, M., Barnekow, A., and Anders, A.,** *Xiphophorus* as an *in vivo* model for studies on normal and defective control of oncogenes, *Adv. Cancer Res.,* 42, 191, 1984.
12. **Anders, F., Schmidt, C.-R., Herbert, A., and Anders, A.,** Prüfung von Kanzerogenen auf Initiator- und/oder Promoteraktivität im Testsystem *Xiphophorus* (Zahnkarpfen), in *Prüfung von Chemikalien auf Cancerogenität, Mutagenität und Teratogenität,* Parchwitz, E., Ed., Gesellschaft f. Strahlenund Umweltforschung, München, 1983, 253.
13. **Barnekow, A. and Gessler, M.,** Activation of $pp60^{c\text{-}src}$ kinase during differentiation of monomyelocytic cells *in vitro, EMBO J.,* 5, 701, 1986.
14. **Barnekow, A., Schartl, M., Anders, F., and Bauer, H.,** Identification of a fish protein associated with a kinase activity and related to the Rous sarcoma virus transforming protein, *Cancer Res.,* 42, 2429, 1982.
15. **Berridge, M. J. and Irvine, R. F.,** Inositol phosphates and cell signalling, *Nature (London),* 341, 197, 1989.

16. **Berridge, M. J.**, Inositol lipids and cell proliferation, *Biochim. Biophys. Acta,* 907, 33, 1987.
17. **Berridge, M. J., Dawson, R. M. C., Downes, C. P., Heslop, J. P., and Irvine, R. F.**, Changes in the levels of inositol phosphates after agonist-dependent hydrolysis of membrane phosphoinositides, *Biochem. J.*, 212, 473, 1983.
18. **Carter, H. R. and Smith, A. D.**, Resolution of the phosphoinositide — specific phospholipase C isolated from porcine lymphocytes into multiple species, *Biochem. J.*, 244, 639, 1987.
19. **Cocco, L., Gilmour, R. S., Ognibene, A., Letcher, A. J., Manzoli, F. A., and Irvine, R. F.**, Synthesis of polyphosphoinositides in nuclei of friend cells, *Biochem. J.*, 248, 765, 1987.
20. **Collet, M. S., Purchio, A. F., and Erikson, R. L.**, Avian sarcoma virus-transforming protein, $pp60^{c\text{-}src}$, shows protein kinase activity specific for tyrosine, *Nature (London),* 285, 167, 1980.
21. **Courtneidge, S. A. and Heber, A.**, An 81 kd protein complexed with middle T antigen and $pp60^{c\text{-}src}$: a possible phosphatidylinositol kinase, *Cell,* 50, 1031, 1987.
22. **Diehl, P.**, Promotions- und Initiationswirkung männlicher und weiblicher Sexualhormone auf die Melanombildung bei ausgewählten *Xiphophorus* -Genotypen, Diplom thesis, University of Giessen, 1986.
23. **Diringer, H. and Friis, R. R.**, Changes in phosphatidylinositol metabolism correlated to growth state of normal and Rous sarcoma virus-transformed Japanese quail cells, *Cancer Res.*, 37, 2979, 1977.
24. **Gordon, M.**, The melanoma cell as an incompletely differentiated pigment cell, in *Pigm. Cell Biol.*, Gordon, M., Ed., Academic Press, New York, 1959, 215.
25. **Hepler, J. R., Nakahata, N., Lovenberg, T. W., DiGuiseppi, J., Herman, B., Earp, H. S., and Harden, T. K.**, Epidermal growth factor stimulates the rapid accumulation of inositol (1,4,5)-triphosphoate and a rise in cytosolic calcium mobilized from intracellular stores in A 431 cells, *J. Biol. Chem.*, 262, 2951, 1987.
26. **Jolles, J., Zwiers, H., Dekker, A., Wirtz, K. W. A., and Gispen, W. H.**, Corticotropin-(1,24)-tetracosapeptide affects protein phosphorylation and polyphosphoinositide metabolism in rat brain, *Biochem. J.*, 194, 283, 1981.
27. **Kaplan, D. R., Whitman, M., Schaffhausen, B., Pallas, D. C., White, M., Cantley, L., and Roberts, T. M.**, Common elements in growth factor stimulation and oncogenic transformation: 85 kd phosphoprotein and phosphatidylinositol kinase activity, *Cell,* 50, 1021, 1987.
28. **Katan, M. and Parker, P. J.**, Oncogenes and cell control, *Nature (London),* 332, 203, 1988.
29. **Katan, M., Kriz, R. W., Totty, N., Philip, R., Meldrum, E., Aldape, R. A., Knopf, S. L., and Parker, P. J.**, Determination of the primary structure of PLC-154 demonstrates diversity of phosphoinositide-specific phospholipase C activities, *Cell,* 54, 171, 1988.
30. **Kersten, H., Schachner, E., Dess, G., Anders, A., Nishimura, S., and Shindo-Okada, N.**, Queuosine in transfer-RNA in relation to differentiation and pteridine metabolism, in *Biochemical and Clinical Aspects of Pteridines,* 2. Curtius, H. Ch., Pfleiderer, W., Wachter, H., Eds., Walter de Gruyter, Berlin, 1983, 367.
31. **Mäueler, W.**, Untersuchungen zur tumorspezifischen Genexpresion bei *Xiphophorus,* Expression von Proto-Onkogenen, Ph.D. thesis, University of Giessen, 1988.
32. **Mäueler, W., Raulf, F., and Schartl, M.**, Expression of proto-oncogenes in embryonic, adult, and transformed tissue of *Xiphophorus* (Teleostei: Poeciliidae), *Oncogene,* 2, 421, 1988.
33. **Mayer, B. J., Hamaguchi, M., and Hanafusa, H.**, A novel viral oncogene with structural similarity to phospholipase C, *Nature (London),* 332, 272, 1988.
34. **Bannasch, P., Griesemer, R. A., Anders, F., Becker, R., Cabral, J. R., and Della Porta, G.**, Assays for initiating and promoting activities, in *Long-Term and Short-Term Assays for Carcinogens: A Critical Appraisal,* Montesano, R., Barth, H., Vainio, H., Wilborn, J., and Yamasaki, H., Eds., IARC Scientific Publications, No. 83, Lyon, 1986, 103.
35. **Pike, L. J. and Eakes, A. T.**, Epidermal growth factor stimulates the production of phosphatidylinositol monophosphate and the breakdown of polyphosphoinositides in A 431 cells, *J. Biol. Chem.*, 262, 1644, 1987.
36. **Pröfrock, A.**, Untersuchungen zum Phosphatidylinosit-Turnover an ausgewählten *Xiphophorus* -Genotypen, Diplom thesis, University of Giessen, 1988.
37. **Ritter, S., Henze, M., and Anders, F.**, Effect of pteridines on normal and neoplastic cell lines of *Xiphophorus, Cell Biol. Int. Rep.*, 12, 431, 1988.
38. **Rozengurt, E.**, Early signals in the mitogenic response, *Science,* 234, 161, 1986.
39. **Schartl, A.**, Modulation der Pigmentzelldifferenzierung durch Sexualsteroide bei *Xiphophorus* und *Girardinus* (Poeciliidae), Ph.D. thesis, University of Giessen, 1988.
40. **Schartl, A., Schartl, M., and Anders, F.**, Promotion and regression of neoplasia by testosterone-promoted cell differentiation in *Xiphophorus* and *Girardinus, Carcinogenesis,* 7, 427, 982.
41. **Schartl, M. and Barnekow, A.**, Differential expression of the cellular *src* gene during vertebrate development, *Dev. Biol.*, 205, 415, 1984.

42. **Schartl, M., Barnekow, A., Bauer, H., and Anders, F.,** Correlations of inheritance and expression between a tumor gene and the cellular homolog of Rous sarcoma virus-transforming gene in *Xiphophorus, Cancer Res.*, 42, 4222, 1982.
43. **Schartl, M., Schmidt, C.-R., Anders, A., and Barnekow, A.,** Elevated expression of the cellular *src* gene in tumors of differing etiology in *Xiphophorus, Int. J. Cancer,* 36, 199, 1985.
44. **Schleenbecker, U.,** Molekulare Analyse zellulärer Gene, die für Wachstumsfaktoren und Wachstumsfaktorrezeptoren kodieren — Untersuchungen an *Xiphophorus* (Pisces; Teleostei), Ph.D. thesis, University of Giessen, 1988.
45. **Stahl, M. L., Ferenz, C. R., Kelleher, K. L., Kriz, R. W., and Knopf, J. L.,** Sequence similarity of phospholipase C with the non-catalytic region of *src, Nature (London),* 332, 269, 1988.
46. **Stich, H. F. and Anders, F.,** The involvement of reactive oxygen species in oral cancers of betel quid/ tobacco chewers, *Mutat. Res.*, 214, 47, 1988.
47. **Sugimoto, Y., Whitman, M., Cantley, L. C., and Erikson, R. L.,** Evidence that the Rous sarcoma virus transforming gene product phosphorylates phosphatidylinositol and diacylglycerol, *Proc. Natl. Acad. Sci. U.S.A.*, 81, 2117, 1984.
48. **Thompson, D. M., Procker, S., Grant, M., and Thomas, C.,** Epidermal growth factor stimulates phosphatidylinositol turnover for ten hours in A 431 cells without activation of protein kinase C, *Biochem. Biophys. Res. Commun.*, 155, 877, 1988.
49. **Vielkind, U.,** Genetic control of cell differentiation in platyfish-swordtail melanomas, *J. Exp. Zool.*, 196, 197, 1976.
50. **Wahl, M. I., Sweatt, J. D., and Carpenter, G.,** Epidermal growth factor (EGF) stimulates inositol triphosphate formation in cells which overexpress the EGF receptor, *Biochem. Biophys. Res. Commun.*, 142, 688, 1987.
51. **Whitman, M., Downes, Cp., Keeler, M., Keller, T., and Cantley, L.,** Type I phosphatidylinositol kinase makes a novel inositol phospholipid, phosphatidylinositol-3-phosphate, *Nature (London),* 332, 644, 1988.
52. **Zechel, Ch., Schleenbecker, U., Anders, A., and Anders, F.,** v-*erb*B related sequences in *Xiphophorus* that map to melanoma determining Mendelian loci and overexpress in a melanoma cell line, *Oncogene,* 3, 605, 1988.
53. **Zechel, Ch., Schleenbecker, U., Anders, A., and Anders, F.,** Regulation of gene expression in the Gordon-Kosswig melanoma system — Approach to study genes involved in the first step to neoplasia, in *New Trends in Ichthyology,* Schröder, H. J., Ed., Paray-Verlag, Hamburg, Berlin, in press, 1989a.
54. **Zechel, Ch., Schleenbecker, U., Anders, A., Pfütz, M., and Anders, F.,** Search for genes critical for the early and/or late events in carcinogenesis: studies in *Xiphophorus* (Pisces, Teleostei), in *Modern Trends in Human Leukemia,* Vol. 8, Neth, R., Ed., Springer-Verlag, Berlin, 1989b.

EPILOGUE

The incidence of maligant melanoma is rapidly increasing in certain sunny geographic areas of the world which have large numbers of immigrant Caucasians. The genetic makeup of some subgroups of Caucasians appears to have a high risk for cutaneous malignant melanoma as a result of the recent cultural change in our outdoor sports and recreational activities. Thus, it would appear that recently altered environmental interaction on long established genetic characteristics of Caucasians has caused a sudden profound increase in the incidence of malignant melanoma. By the year 2000, we will have an epidemic of CMM that will affect 1 in 100 Caucasians.

We have provided a clinicopathologic and genetic survey of primarily the most common of the hereditary malignant malanomas, namely, the familial atypical multiple mole melanoma (FAMMM) syndrome. The FAMMM syndrome has and can serve as a model for clinical and basic research in cancer genetics. Though this review has been broad in its scope and has illuminated the different facets of the FAMMM syndrome, it has been more revealing in the demonstration of our lack of knowledge of the etiology and pathogenesis of this cancer associated genodermatosis. The FAMMM genotype may be a very significant factor in the melanoma upsurge we are now experiencing.

We have established the autosomal dominance of the FAMMM syndrome but we have not established the extent of the heterogeneity of the disease. We still have to define the spectrum of the phenotypic variation of the cutaneous phenotypes of atypical nevi and the number of moles needed to establish the diagnosis of the FAMMM syndrome. It is apparent that not all FAMMM kindreds have the same risk for malignant melanoma; however, are the genotypes of the FAMMM syndrome the same in different tribal groups of Caucasians? Investigators have confused the issue of sporadic occurrence of the atypical nevus so that the data now available are so inadequate historically that new in-depth investigations will have to be done to clarify these concerns. It is essential that the old mistakes of lack of genetic investigations not be repeated and that these inquiries use medical and pathologic records for confirmation of all data be they negative or positive.

There is no doubt that we now recognize the florid extreme of the cutaneous phenotypes, but we do not even perceive the more subtle facets of the FAMMM clinical spectrum. What are the minimal characteristics of atypical nevi with respect to size, irregularity of border, color variation, contour changes, and number? Are atypical nevi found in normal persons and with what frequency? When does the absence of atypical nevi in a patient rule out the presence of the FAMMM genotype? Are the total number of moles a better indicator of the genotypic status than the presence of atypical nevi? Thus, our clinical investigations of the phenotypic expression of the heterogeneity of the FAMMM syndrome have just begun.

Normally, the histologic interpretation of tissue has given some sense of security to the diagnosis of a clinical state. In the case of the dysplastic nevus, histologic interpretations have led to more problems than they have solved. The minimal histologic definition of dysplastic nevi has not clearly separated normal nevi from the pathologic state. We will have to address the issue of the minimal histologic characteristics of dysplastic nevi. At the other end of the histologic spectrum is the difficulty of interpreting the distinction of dysplastic nevi from melanoma *in situ*. We will also have to address the issue of histologically confirmed atypical nevi in normal persons. Are dysplastic nevi normal nevi in a very active metabolic state which we cannot classify as either normal or abnormal? It may well be that the limits will never be precise, and we will have to add ancillary biological testing methods to establish the clinical diagnosis.

The concept of the FAMMM syndrome as a cancer-associated genodermatosis has implications of high risk for malignant melanoma and also in some FAMMM kindreds, there appear to be integral patterns of systemic cancers. These phenomena have placed this syndrome in accord with the usual pattern of the cancer-associated genodermatoses; that is, the risk for cancer involves many organ systems with an excess of multiple primary malignant neoplasms. More research will be required to elucidate the heterogeneity of this aspect of the syndrome. In order for cost-effective cancer surveillance programs to be established, we must be able to identify the particular pattern of systemic cancer for those FAMMM families who are at high risk for systemic cancer. It is here that genetic linkage analysis, along with biomolecular and cytogenetic studies may be most useful in identifying those kindreds at greatest cancer risk for multiple organ systems.

Is controversy in science good? Historically, it has provided the stimulus to solve the complex problems unearthed by inquiry. What is needed is continued, systematic research in many disciplines (e.g., epidemiological, genetic, clinical, histologic, and biomolecular), but especially in gene linkage and cancer biomarkers with the objective of achieving acceptable sensitivity and specificity for the FAMMM genotype. Ongoing efforts in cytogenetics showing chromosome breakage and specific translocations in the FAMMM syndrome should lead to invaluable clues towards the attainment of these objectives. A flowering of research by different groups around the world should be encouraged even though their concepts may be in conflict.

Thus, more funding is needed to support these research efforts if we are to attain our goal of reversing the trend of increasing occurrence of malignant melanoma, which by the year 2000, will affect 1 in 100 Caucasians. We are anticipating the opportunity to provide a future edition in which we may be able to elucidate further this entire issue of hereditary malignant melanoma.

INDEX

N

O

P